Activities Handbook and Instructor's Guide for *Expanding Options for Older Adults with Developmental Disabilities*

A Practical Guide to Achieving Community Access

Also available is **Expanding Options for Older Adults with Developmental Disabilities: A Practical Guide to Achieving Community Access.** To order this text, contact Paul H. Brookes Publishing Co., P. O. Box 10624, Baltimore, MD 21285-0624.

Activities Handbook and Instructor's Guide for *Expanding Options for Older Adults with Developmental Disabilities*

A Practical Guide to Achieving Community Access

by

Marion Stroud, Ph.D.
Director of Research and Development

and

Evelyn Sutton, M.A.
Gerontology Consultant

ACCESS: Cooperative Planning
for Services to Aged Persons
with Developmental
Disabilities
The University of Akron
Akron, Ohio

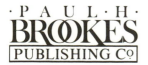
·P·A·U·L·H·
BROOKES
PUBLISHING CO.

Baltimore · London · Toronto · Sydney

Paul H. Brookes Publishing Co.
Post Office Box 10624
Baltimore, Maryland 21285-0624

Typeset by Brushwood Graphics Inc., Baltimore, Maryland.
Manufactured in the United States of America by
The Maple Press Company, York, Pennsylvania.

Original photographs by Christine Cikra.

Library of Congress Cataloging-in-Publication Data
Stroud, Marion, 1922–
    Activities handbook and instructor's guide for expanding options for
older adults with developmental disabilities.

    1. Developmentally disabled aged—Rehabilitation—Study and teach-
ing.   2. Developmentally disabled aged—Rehabilitation.   3. Develop-
mentally disabled aged—Life skills guides.   I. Sutton, Evelyn.
II. Title.
HV1570.S76   1988   362.1′968   88-6137
ISBN 0-933716-94-X (pbk.)

Contents

How to Use This Book

WHO   The Activities Handbook is to be used by staff of agencies that serve developmentally disabled older adults, whether in special services for them or in generic community services they attend.

The Instructor's Guide is to be used by staff development trainers in these agencies. The materials also were developed for use by and with families and advocates of older adults with developmental disabilities.

HOW   Both parts of this book can be read for information and kept as a ready reference. It is not necessary that trainees memorize all information contained in the Instructor's Guide, but only that they meet the objectives listed in training and know how to locate needed information in the book.

TRAINING   The instructor can select from the Activities Handbook the lessons needed by the trainees. Ideally, this is done on the basis of the results of a pretest, but selection can also be made by trainees who indicate their own needs. Each lesson is designed for about 1 hour of presentation time if the activities are included. The total presentation time could be 6 hours if the instructor covered every lesson. In the field test presentations of this material, the time varied from a 1-hour overview to a full day of in-service.

Each lesson plan in the Instructor's Guide is designed to be presented in about 1 hour. This allows for lecture and discussion, as well as for participation in an activity to reinforce the learning. The plans can be adapted to meet the special needs of each group. The authors found that some audiences already had basic information about developmental disabilities, while others knew about aging. In these cases, the instructor emphasized information about the area less well known. Total presentation time in the field testing ranged from a 2-hour overview to full-day in-services.

FORMAT   The Activities Handbook contains lessons grouped into seven areas of competence: grooming/health, clothing, social interaction, personal security, community activities, public transportation, and leisure/recreational activities. Each activity in these lessons is designed to give trainees experience in the skills of daily living, self-help, and communication that are necessary for maximizing their ability to access community services.

Each lesson in the Instructor's Guide consists of a lesson plan with objectives, instructor's activities, learner activities, materials, and evaluation. Lecture outlines are provided as needed, and the activities are presented for duplication as handouts.

Activities Handbook and Instructor's Guide for *Expanding Options for Older Adults with Developmental Disabilities*

A Practical Guide to Achieving Community Access

PART 1

Activities Handbook

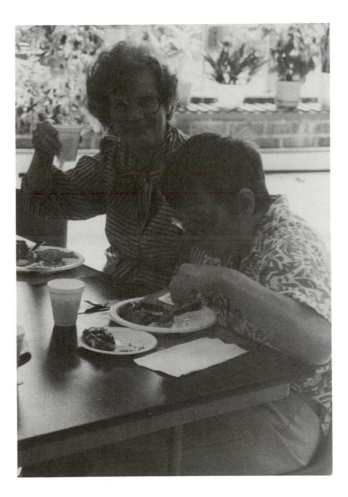

Introduction

Successful inclusion of developmentally disabled older adults in community services is the focus of *Expanding Options for Older Adults with Developmental Disabilities*. Each step toward that goal brings closer the time when older adults with disabilities will be able to anticipate retirement; then they may enjoy new activities in the company of the citizens of the community, doing new things, going places, making friends, and making the most of that time of life.

CHARACTERISTICS OF OLDER ADULTS WITH MR/DD

ACCESS research into the characteristics of about 100 older adults in Northeastern Ohio showed that about three fourths of these people were good candidates for participation in community activities. Most of them were in good health, ambulatory, independent in self-care skills, and able to get along well with others.

Historically, almost all had been institutionalized for part or most of their lives, since that was the accepted treatment during their youth. Few had any formal education, and so they were unable to read or write or use money. Most of them had been active, were well nourished, kept regular hours, and received medical attention, however.

Institutional life had the effect of depriving them of experiences common to most of the population. They did not have lasting personal relationships and did not marry or have children to raise. Most of them worked on the grounds of the institution and never experienced competitive employment. Their lives were relatively free of the stresses most people face, but the richness of relationships and excitements of ordinary living were missed.

When they were interviewed by the researchers, many said that they wished they had someone to care about them, some special friend. Because there are many changes of staff and residents in an institution, residents learn that it is best not to care too much about anyone since they will probably not be around for long. Institutional living does not foster development of the social skills needed for interaction with residents of the community.

TRAINING NEEDS

Training needs of developmentally disabled older adults who could be integrated into community services were identified in the ACCESS study. These included:

1. Dressing and grooming for different occasions. How to decide what type of occasion and setting will be encountered, and how to choose clothing similar to that which others will be wearing.
2. How to use prosthetics properly. The importance of wearing one's dentures and hearing aid. How to keep teeth and mouth clean and sweet-smelling. How to use dental adhesives or get painful dentures fixed.
3. Increasing social interaction skills, such as how to carry on casual conversations, how to participate in activities with nonretarded people, how to play table games, how to behave at a performance, and especially, what is and is not appropriate to discuss with others.

4. How to relate to another person without becoming too dependent on that person for all approval and social contact. How to control too much telephoning or personal encounters.

5. Knowing what to do when one is lost or confused or in trouble. Knowing how to ask for assistance, what information one needs to be able to provide, how to use a telephone, and who to call for help.

6. Expanding the mental environment of clients by increasing their knowledge of the world in which they live. This includes knowing the geography of the community, what services and activities are available there, how to access them, and what expectations of others need to be accommodated.

7. How to use public transportation—buses if they are available, or taxis. How to give directions and how to pay.

These training needs are addressed in an outline format in this book and are organized according to the areas of training required by many agencies for the convenience of the interdisciplinary teams: self-help skills (grooming/health), daily living skills (clothing, personal security, community activities, public transportation), leisure/recreational activities, and communication skills (social interaction).

TRAINING IN SOCIAL SKILLS

Before beginning a training program it is important to know whether the trainee is likely to be able to learn the behaviors and information presented. Fortunately, there is a strong background of research in this area that indicates that people with developmental disabilities can learn social skills.

Research in training individuals with developmental disabilities in social skills is extensive. Davies and Rogers[1] reported on 31 studies done between 1967 and 1984. Motoric-physical behaviors learned by the individuals included social greeting, smiling, physical contact, decreasing negative behaviors, positive prosocial interaction, and verbal interaction. Social skills and behaviors learned included assertiveness, expression of praise and appreciation, conversing, making small talk, asking for help, disagreeing, social rituals, personal appearance, and making friends. Social-cognitive skills included role taking, referential thinking, consequential thinking in interpersonal encounters, and self-monitoring strategies. An excellent reference list of the studies is included in the article by Davies and Rogers. Those who are planning training activities will find it a useful resource for preparatory reading.

Davies and Rogers[1] listed the training methods that were successful with the MR/DD population. Direct teaching, physical and verbal prompting, shaping, modeling, and coaching all produced learning. The most frequently used and successful methods were *visual modes of instruction, practice, and contingent reinforcement.*

Generalization of the learned skills into other settings is less often studied. It is generally acknowledged that individuals with developmental disabilities need to practice learned skills in the settings where they will be used. Simulations and role plays may demonstrate strategies for interaction to the trainees, but these strategies must be practiced over and over in the places where they will be used. For example, a person may learn how to simulate giving destinations to a taxi driver, or carrying on conversations about the weather, but when confronted with the real situation he or she may forget the skill entirely. Therefore, it is important to plan for generalization of learning by practicing the skills in the community where they will be used. This might be accomplished by enlisting the cooperation of others, such as interested nonhandicapped people at a senior center or a volunteer escort who would accompany the trainee to a community activity and remain available to advise or help if needed.

Davies and Rogers[1] recommend some important considerations for those who are developing training programs. They are summarized here:

1. Comprehensive, technically accurate curricula for training in social skills need to be developed.
2. Visual instruction, active rehearsal, and practice are the most effective methods of instruction.
3. New skills should be contingently reinforced.
4. The newly learned skills should be applied in the environment where they will be used.
5. Evaluate the results of training in terms of the client's improved social life.
6. Study the relationship between the individual's intellectual abilities and the acquisition of social skills.

ACCESS TRAINING METHODS

ACCESS training methods are discussed in Section III in the primary text. These suggestions are repeated here:

Work toward specific objectives: Adults who are motivated by the prospect of new opportunities for recreation and social contacts need goal-directed activities in preparation for the experience.

Vary the mode of teaching: Avoid too much talking or lecturing. Add depth to learning activities with pictures, slides, films, tapes, and real materials. Whenever possible, let the learner do the talking, modeling, role play, videotaping, and other aspects of the activity that require involvement.

Provide for practice: Repeat the learning activity and gradually increase the reality level. Practice can extend to a dress rehearsal just before going into the community. Be sure to provide support for the learner during the first times the skill is used in public.

Don't expect perfection: Developmentally disabled older adults do not have to measure up to some standard for senior citizens in order to participate in community programs. The purpose of advance preparation is to minimize embarrassment and frustration, and to ensure comfortable and pleasant experiences in the company of others.

Provide for friends or escorts to accompany the older adult to new places and remain available until a comfort level is established: Everyone feels a bit shy when encountering new situations, and for the inexperienced older adult with DD this can be a real stumbling block.

Utilize volunteers to expand the opportunities for community access: Successful integration is most likely to succeed if one client goes with one escort. Every effort should be made to avoid sending large groups of MR/DD adults into a community site.

TEACHING MODES

Show, Don't Tell

Marc Gold's[2] well-known system of instruction in work skills, "Try Another Way," emphasizes that developmentally disabled people are likely to have difficulty interpreting a stream of talk directed at them while they are learning. Gold observed that individuals could learn best with a minimum of verbal instruction, especially during the practice period. He suggested silent demonstration of the desired behaviors and limited instructors to one or two words or short, repeated phrases while the trainee was working on the task.

Slow thinkers need to be given time to solve problems. Often the leader will wait only a second or two before giving verbal prompts or answers to questions. Give plenty of time for trainees to figure out what to do or say; otherwise they will learn to wait long enough for you to do it for them.

The leader should consistently use the same words for things so that the trainee can respond without having to think about what is meant. For example, in teaching clients to give the destination to a driver, always use the same words, "Tell where you are going" instead of sometimes saying, "Give him the address" or "Say the place you want." This isn't an iron-clad rule; it simply makes instruction less confusing for the learner.

Ginott[3] advises instructors to be careful of how they talk to learners in order to keep personal references to a minimum. Talk about the problem, not the person: "Give him the address," not "You have to remember to tell the driver the address. Don't forget it like you always do." The second message has a put-down in it that will be louder than the instruction.

Model Behaviors, Don't Describe Them

Dreikurs, Grunwald, and Pepper[4] define modeling as "teaching through example that produces learning through imitation." Behaviors to be learned are modeled or acted out while the adults watch carefully. The model may be the leader or another adult. After watching the behavior once or twice, the group might discuss what was done and what effect it had on each of the participants. Then volunteers from the group could try to demonstrate the behaviors and have their efforts critiqued by the whole group. Finally, every member of the learning group could model either the precise behavior or an application of it in a different setting.

Models do not have to be live performances by people. Tapes, records, photographs, or objects can be used effectively. Videotapes are very effective to use in modeling because the exact behavior and setting can be reproduced, and the tape can be viewed immediately and as often as desired. Sound is also recorded automatically. Use of a variety of modes encourages repeated use by trainees.

Small Group Work

Training programs for developmentally disabled people tend to focus almost entirely on individual instruction because of the individualized habilitation plan (IHP) required for each client. However, some skills are best developed in group work. The best practice of interaction skills comes in real situations where the reactions of others cannot be anticipated, but must be dealt with as they occur.

In habilitation classes or residential programs small group formation is one way of providing clients the experience of *belonging*. The group can form lasting friendships in which they are able to care for each other and feel attachment to the group. One such group of older adults with retardation exchanges birthday cards, gifts, and telephone calls, and shares activities that bind the members of the group to each other in ways they have not previously experienced.

The activities suggested here often include discussion questions for small groups. The leader can propose the question and clarify it, but then should wait until the members respond. Again, it is important for the leader to avoid doing the talking. Most of the members of the group will have had many years experience letting others talk *for* them. It is hard at first for everyone to sit through long periods of silence, but the members need time to unlearn the passive reactions that have served them well for so long.

The leader can reinforce responses by listing the ideas on a blackboard or chart as they are given by trainees. Even if they can't read, members will note that their response is valued. The written responses can be read back to the group to encourage additional comments and to summarize at the end of the discussion.

Group meetings can also be helpful in teaching problem solving and decision making. The leader's role should not be manipulative. Glasser[5] stresses the importance of the leader's commitment to having the members develop strength and independence. The leader makes a conscious effort not to influence the discussion unduly by making suggestions before the members have had time to think, or advocating solutions before they have been considered. When the leader takes over and does all the thinking and talking, the members soon learn to be passive and not participate. Such experiences encourage dependence rather than foster learning.

Group meetings are supposed to focus on problem solving and should never be allowed to become gripe sessions or attacks on personalities. The leader can demonstrate how to solve problems by structuring the thinking. Gordon's[6] No-Lose method of resolving problems has these steps that can be used in small group work:

1. Define the problem
2. Generate possible solutions
3. Evaluate the solutions
4. Decide which solution is best
5. Determine how to implement the solution
6. Assess how well the solution solved the problem

As the members discuss the pros and cons of each alternative, they are involved in decision making and have a commitment to making the solution work.

SOME CAUTIONS

Leaders must be sensitive to possible hidden messages that might be inadvertently conveyed to developmentally disabled adults when they are getting ready to access community activities. They may get the impression that everyone will be looking at them, judging every move, criticizing the way they look and act. Such fears will spoil the fun of going new places and meeting new people.

The purpose of the training activities is to decrease the elements of strangeness in new settings. If the participants know that they look like others, know how to do the activities, know how to carry on simple conversations, and know they will not be different, they can concentrate on enjoying the new experiences.

Positive reinforcement of desired behaviors is a key concept of all instructional programs for MR/DD persons. Age-appropriate social reinforcers are well used to encourage learning of needed skills for community access. Praise, recognition, being chosen to demonstrate a skill to others, applause—all are age appropriate. The ultimate reinforcer should be actual participation in the activity being studied. Negatives should be especially avoided because they will convey the hidden messages that take the fun out of going out and set the client up for failure.

DO IT YOURSELF

The activities presented here are in a format that the leader can follow in designing other learning experiences. The format generally includes the following pattern of elements:

1. Motivate—relate the new activity to something known from a previous experience, to a television show, to a trip taken, to a familiar person.
2. Employ visual presentation—use pictures, slides, photos, real objects such as products, different kinds of foods, tools, charts, exhibits. Whenever possible have the members of the group arrange or present.
3. Interpret and teach—guide the members in learning the skill. Use modeling if possible.
4. Provide practice—allow members to demonstrate skills, go at their own speed, get lots of encouragement, role play, or work in pairs. When they feel ready, they may be video- or audiotaped for their own critique.
5. Reinforce—give members opportunities to use the new skill. Learning is generalized and reinforced by practicing the skill in the setting where it will be used.
6. Give alternatives—provide variations on the activity to show that there are a number of possibilities for enjoyment of the new interest.

REFERENCES

1. Davies, R. R., & Rogers, E. A. (1985). Social skills training with persons who are mentally retarded. *Mental Retardation, 23*(4), 186–195.
2. Gold, M. (1975). *Try another way.* Indianapolis, IN: Film Productions of Indianapolis. [Film]
3. Ginott, J. (1972). *Teacher and child: A book for parents and teachers.* New York: Macmillan.
4. Dreikurs, R., Grunwald, B., & Pepper, F. (1971). *Maintaining sanity in the classroom.* New York: Harper & Row.
5. Glasser, W. (1965). *Reality therapy: A new approach to psychiatry.* New York: Harper & Row.
6. Gordon, T. (1977). *TET: Teacher effectiveness training.* New York: McKay.

Training Activities

GROOMING/HEALTH (SELF-HELP)

Unit I. Appearance/Cleanliness

Lesson A: Knowing How You Look _____

Objectives

1. To be able to recognize one's face
2. To be able to recognize others from photos
3. To know details about one's appearance

Activities

1. Provide each person or small group with a fairly large hand mirror. Have each person examine face carefully and be ready to tell the color of hair and eyes and shape of face.
2. Find another person in the group who has the same colors. Learn the names for hair colors (e.g., blonde, brunette, grey, white).
3. Take several photos of each member of the group. One should show the face in close-up. Another should show full body front view. The third photo should show a side view.
4. Have the participants mount the pictures on cardboard and write their names below the photos. Make a gallery of group pictures to use in other activities.
5. Using catalogues or colored advertisements from the newspaper, have clients cut out pictures of people with the same hair and eye colors as their own, and, if possible, people with the same general body type. Paste these on paper and write "Look-alike" under each picture with the name of the person it resembles.

Variations

1. As activities in the community are being considered, add to the gallery photos of people from the new setting.
2. When speakers or guests come to give presentations to the group, take their pictures to add to the gallery.
3. Add photos of day program staff to the gallery.

Materials

1. Large hand mirror for each participant
2. Camera and film
3. Catalogues, color advertisement sections from newspapers
4. Cardboard, railway board, or construction paper and glue

Lesson B: Hand Awareness —————————————————————————

Objectives

1. To know what one's hands look like
2. To know some ways to make hands more attractive to others

Activities

1. Each client looks at hands and is ready to report on such things as length of fingernails, cleanliness, rings, and so forth.
2. Women note whether they are wearing nail polish and, if so, what condition it is in.
3. Men note condition of nails, whether filed evenly, cuticle.
4. Display hand care products, lotions, heavy-duty cleansers, soaps, nail polishes, removers, nail files, emery boards, cuticle sticks. Discuss and demonstrate use of each —give time for clients to try the products.
5. Display variety of nail polish colors. Let clients try the brightest and wildest and the simplest clear ones. Discuss occasions when each is appropriate/inappropriate.
6. Discuss the effects of various kinds of weather on the hands. What precautions are needed to avoid chapped hands in winter? How do lotions and gloves protect?

Variations

1. Display gloves as accessories, gloves for protection, work gloves, and so forth
2. Have a volunteer give each member of the group a manicure using soapy soak, buffing, emery board, and cuticle stick.
3. Advertisements for nail products can be cut out and mounted to show well-cared-for hands, nail polish colors, or lotions.
4. Show display of different kinds of rings that can be worn; possibly borrow from accessory store. Cut out pictures of rings from jewelry catalogue.

Materials

1. Nail care products—emery boards, nail files, cuticle sticks, and so forth
2. Hand care products—soaps, heavy-duty cleaners, lotions
3. Gloves—accessories, protective
4. Ring display or pictures from catalogues

Lesson C: Hair Care _____

Objectives

1. To know what type and color of hair one has
2. To be able to use hair care products
3. To know what hairstyles are becoming and how to achieve them
4. To be able to shampoo and groom hair

Activities

1. Using the photo of self from the gallery, look at the hair color and recall the name of the color for each client.
2. Decide what hairstyle each person had: permed, short cut, waved, long, etc.
3. How are hairstyles maintained? Does one go to barber or hairdresser? Discuss frequency of service and cost.
4. Display hair care products and explain use of each: shampoo, conditioner, color, brushes, combs, curlers, setting lotion, hair spray.
5. Demonstrate correct way to shampoo, rinse, and dry. If hair is set, show how that is done; if a curling iron is used, demonstrate how to do it safely.
6. Discuss hair grooming in public. Discuss expectations of others that hair will be combed not in public, but in restrooms or where others will not see it.

Variations

1. Invite a hairdresser to demonstrate hair styling.
2. Use magazines and group discussion to select the hairstyles "best for me."
3. Visit a school for cosmetologists.

Materials

1. Hair care products: combs, brushes, shampoos, conditioners, spray, curlers, setting lotions
2. Photos of each client from the gallery
3. Pictures of different hairstyles from magazines

Lesson D: Dental Self-Examination

Objectives

1. To be aware of how teeth look and most attractive way to smile
2. To be able to care for teeth and use products effectively
3. To be able to care for dentures

Activities

1. Have clients use large hand mirrors to examine their teeth to know exactly how they appear to others. Look at the face with the mouth closed and then smiling. Look at all kinds of ways of smiling: wide mouth (showing the teeth) and closed mouth. Decide which looks best and practice it.
2. Display various kinds of toothbrushes and toothpastes or cleaners. Discuss the advantages of each: brushes designed to clean under the gums, round brushes, hard or medium bristles; cleaners that whiten teeth, those that protect against cavities, those for smokers.
3. Review the right way to clean teeth and mouth, giving each person a chance to demonstrate if desired.
4. For clients with dentures, discuss the importance of wearing dentures for chewing food and getting it ready to digest. Discuss the effect of wearing dentures on appearance. (This should be done one-on-one to prevent embarrassment.) Be sure to compliment them when they do wear their dentures.
   • If dentures are not comfortable, discuss the need to give that information to staff so that a dentist can be consulted. Emphasize the importance of wearing the dentures in public, especially since others judge one by appearance.
   • Use of adhesives for dentures can be demonstrated and practiced. Have the denture wearer watch commercials for the various brands and comment on what the maker says each one will do. Bring in several brands for testing. Denture cleaners can be tested in class; try using chalk as is done in commercials.

Variations

1. Cut out pictures of people who have nice smiles. Make a montage.
2. Cut out advertisements for dental products. Put them on cards to use in identifying those special uses claimed for each.
3. Make a display of dental products with the names of clients who use each one.
4. Invite a dental hygienist to talk to the group and demonstrate oral hygiene.

Materials

1. Hand mirror for each client
2. Various kinds of toothbrushes, toothpastes, cleaners
3. Denture adhesives and cleaners

Lesson E: Care and Appearance of Eyes _____

Objectives

1. To be able to cleanse and care for eyes
2. To know how to use simple eye cosmetics (women)
3. To know how to care for eyeglasses

Activities

1. Display eye care products (eye drops, boric acid, etc.) and discuss their use. Stress that they are not used ordinarily or daily unless so advised by a doctor; they are for occasional use when eyes are strained.
2. Use advertisements from newspapers and magazines; discuss glasses, bifocals, reading glasses, contacts (soft and extended wear).
3. Demonstrate the correct way to clean glasses so they will not be scratched. Show how to put them down so the lens doesn't touch the surface. Emphasize the importance of keeping them in a case when not in use.
4. Explain the importance of having glasses properly seated on the face with all the screws tight and temples over ears.
5. (*Women can do this and men can give opinions.*) Display eye makeup: eye shadows, eyebrow pencils, and powder mascaras. Make up one woman using vivid color and lots of it. Make up another using more natural color and not overdone. Men judge.
6. Women who want to learn how to make up eyes can have a small group to learn and practice. Take "before" and "after" photos.

Variations

1. Ask an optometrist to talk to the class about eye care.
2. Cut out and mount pictures of women with different eye makeup.
3. Group make a videotape of correct way to clean and care for glasses.

Materials

1. Eye care products, eye drops, ointments, and so forth
2. Pictures of different types of eye makeup
3. Cosmetics for eyes: eye shadows, pencils, mascara

Lesson F: Care and Decoration of Ears

Objectives

1. To know some rules for care of ears
2. To know about earrings and be able to select appropriate ones to accessorize outfits
3. To know how to take care of a hearing aid

Activities

1. Discuss prevention of hearing loss. Place radio or tape recorder in center of group. Turn it up very loud. Analyze reactions. Did it hurt? Were you uncomfortable? Does it damage ears? Point out that many young people are losing their hearing because they listen to music too loud for their ears to stand.
2. Discuss care of outer ear. Place objects on table: washcloth, bobby pin, Q-tip, toothpick. Ask which are safe to use to clean ears. The washcloth is the only safe ear-cleaning tool. If earwax accumulates, a doctor can clean it. Do not use any products found at a drugstore.
3. Discuss care of hearing aid. Generally the staff will do the testing to determine the power of the batteries and the working efficiency of the aid. The wearer should limit care to wiping the aid with tissue to prevent the buildup of earwax. The aid should not be washed.
4. Help clients understand hearing loss. Play the radio or spoken tape very softly so that it is hard to understand. Talk to individuals in a low voice, leaving out the "s" sounds. If possible, find a record at a speech clinic that gives the sounds as heard by a person with hearing loss.

    • Pretend to talk to one person using no voice at all while looking at another person as though you were talking about him/her. Laugh and convey the idea that you are really discussing that person. When the target person notices, ask what feelings he felt when he thought he was the subject of conversation but didn't know what was being said. Discuss the idea that hearing problems can lead to people feeling left out, confused, and disliked.
5. Discuss what a hearing aid does. Show a hearing aid to the class or have a client who wears one demonstrate it. Let each person listen to the amplified sound. Point out that the aid does not make sound clearer, only louder.
6. Demonstrate earrings as accessories to make women look more attractive or dressed-up. Place a number of sets of earrings, both pierced and clip style, on a piece of velvet. Have enough clip style earrings that all can try them on. Display the fullest range of styles and types possible.

    • Have the clients try the earrings on themselves and look in the mirror. After a few minutes, ask how their ear lobes feel. Do they hurt? Which styles do they like? Do the long, dangling ones get caught in their collars? Are they heavy? Does anyone want to get ears pierced? Talk about why women go through having their ears pierced (because earrings don't hurt after scar tissue forms; because earrings are less likely to be lost).
7. Cut pictures from magazines, color advertisements, or catalogues showing women wearing various kinds of earrings. Have each person make a collection of pictures showing the kind to wear for daytime activities, those that match outfits, those that just look good with any outfit (gold, silver), and those that are suitable only for special evening dress-up occasions.

    Men should participate in activities 6 and 7 for fun and so that they can get a sense of decision making about appropriate dress for different settings and occasions. Men can act as judges, giving "thumbs up" to combinations they like.

Variations

1. Ask a hearing aid salesperson to talk to the class and display different kinds of aids.
2. Invite the program nurse to tell about ear hygiene.
3. Visit a department store or jewelry store to look at earrings.
4. Collect donated earrings from staff to use as reinforcers and rewards.

Materials

1. Model or chart showing parts of ear
2. Washcloth, bobby pin, Q-tip, toothpick
3. Tape recorder, radio, record player that can be made very loud
4. Big collection of earrings, both pierced and clip-on
5. Large hand mirrors

Lesson G: Care of Feet and Choosing Shoes ————————————

Objectives

1. To know how to care for feet
2. To be able to choose shoes that are comfortable and supporting

Activities

1. Demonstrate on a real foot how to wash feet correctly, especially between the toes, and dry thoroughly.
    *   Discuss importance of wearing something on feet in public showers, as at a swimming pool, to prevent catching athlete's foot.
2. Demonstrate correct trimming of toenails on real foot. Use clippers and scissors.
3. Ask program nurse or a podiatrist to discuss care of blisters, corns, bunions, ingrown toenails, and so forth.
4. In a store, look at display of foot care products. Discuss how they can be used to increase comfort. Look at foam insoles and discuss how they can help feet absorb the pressures of walking.
5. Invite the manager of a shoe store to demonstrate proper fitting of shoes as well as styles that are comfortable for working or walking.
    *   Ask that same person to bring in a variety of styles of shoes so that there are some for special occasions, for sports, for hiking, and other special uses.
6. Cut advertisements for shoes out of magazines, catalogues, and newspapers. Make charts: Work/Sport/Hiking/Party/Church. Place the pictures of shoes under appropriate categories.

Variations

1. Take one or two individuals to shoe stores to be fitted. Be sure they know their size after the clerk measures them.
2. Learn some toe-wiggling foot exercises.

Materials

1. Soap, water, towel
2. Foot remedies from store
3. Magazines, catalogues, newspaper advertisement sections, scissors, paste, mounting paper

Unit II.   Use of Toiletries

Lesson H: Smelling Nice (Deodorants and Scents) _____

Objectives

1. To be able to use deodorants
2. To be able to use scents and scented products

Activities

1. Display deodorants of all kinds and brands: powders, sprays, solids, those for men and those for women. Have each person pick out the kind he/she uses. Let each one in turn demonstrate how to use that kind or brand to the whole group.
2. Introduce scents with some scented items that people buy just to enjoy the scent: scented candles, potpourri, incense, flowers.
   - Show some scented items used to cover up other smells: household sprays, pine-scented cleaners, scented toilet paper, room deodorizers. Let each person smell them as desired.
   - Discuss smells clients like: coffee, food cooking, fresh grass, clean towels. People like things that smell good, clean, delicious.
3. Display soap, talc, after-shave, and cologne for men. Display soap, scented talc, cologne, and perfume for women. Let everyone smell what he/she wants. Put a dab on their hands to smell. Let them notice how the scent changes after it has been on the skin for a while.
   - Demonstrate and discuss where to wear scent, how much is enough, and how often to replace it. Let someone put on too much and/or too many different scents. Let others say how that smells to them.

Variations

1. Invite a sales representative for an inexpensive line of cosmetics to bring in her collection of scents for men and women to demonstrate to class.
2. Ask each member of the group to bring in the kind of scented toiletries he/she uses. Let everyone smell the scent and see if it makes them think of the person who used it.
3. Make a Christmas shopping list of favorite scents to be given as gifts to whom they would be given.

Materials

1. All types of deodorants (spray, solid, powder, for male/female)
2. Scented household products, scented candles, incense, potpourri, flowers
3. Toiletries that are scented, after-shave, cologne, perfume talc

Lesson I: Cosmetics for Older Adults ────────────────

Objectives

1. To know what kind of cosmetics are appropriate for older adults to wear
2. To be able to apply cosmetics correctly

Activities

1. Have clients cut out advertisements of cosmetics for women and men from magazines (use *Esquire* or *Ebony* for men). Mount those that portray adults and fairly conservative makeup. Let clients help with the selection of the appropriate ones.
2. Have the clients bring in the cosmetics they presently use. If the men don't have any, they can either serve as advisers for women or do something else entirely. Let each person demonstrate how each product is applied, and have the others notice the effect. If something more is needed, have it available to try.
3. Make a display of cosmetics for women: makeup base, lipstick, lotion or cream, face powder (if desired), blusher, eye shadow, eyebrow pencil, mascara. Have someone who is skilled in makeup application make up those who wish to try it. Take "before" and "after" pictures.

    Let the group comment on the effects of the makeup. Does it make the person look better, more attractive, younger, healthier? Do they prefer her with little or no makeup. Discuss how it is the person's own decision whether to use it or not. Many women do use makeup and look better in it; others use little or none and look good that way.
4. Men are not expected to use makeup and everyone thinks they look fine without it. Some men use a little cologne and some talc on the face, especially if they have heavy whiskers.

Variations

1. Invite a sales representative for an inexpensive line of cosmetics to come to the group and do some special makeup applications for some of the women.
2. Take the women to a department store to look at all the cosmetics. List the prices of some of the lipsticks, creams, and other cosmetics; then go to an inexpensive variety store and compare prices.

Materials

1. All kinds of makeup cosmetics: lipsticks, eye shadows, mascara, blusher, base, creams, lotions powders
2. Magazines for women and men that have advertisements for cosmetics; scissors and mounting materials

CLOTHING (DAILY LIVING)

Unit III.   Dressing Well

Lesson A: Matching Outfits from What You Have _____

Objectives

1. To be able to select matching outfits from clothing already owned; to know what goes together
2. To be aware of own clothes that do not go together
3. To know what kinds of clothing need to be added so that they will fill needs and be wearable in combination with items in wardrobe

Activities

1. At the residence, working with just two roommates, go through major clothes items in each closet and list by colors: pants, jackets or cardigan sweaters, skirts, suits.

    Place a star (∗) beside those that are for work or day program. Place a circle (○) beside those for sport or active leisure. Place a plus (+) beside those for church or dress occasions.

    • Next, go through the blouses, shirts, and tops, listing the colors and putting the symbol for work, sports, or dress beside each.

    • What are the most common colors in the person's wardrobe? Do wardrobe items have patterns of their own, or are they single colors that go with many other colors?

    Talk with each person about the basic colors and patterns in the main part of the wardrobe. Decide which are most liked, most durable, and most liked by others, and which to build on.

    • Leave the wardrobe list with the person to keep and add to.

2. At the residence, working with roommates, take out a pair of pants belonging to the person; request that a top or shirt that matches or goes with it be chosen (more than one, if possible). Continue this as necessary until the concept of "going together" is clear.

    Select a brightly patterned garment and do the same as above. If the person is confused, offer suggestions of how to match specific colors in the pattern.

    • Place two strongly patterned pieces together and talk about the concept of clashing; or do the same with incompatible colors. Have the person select a plain garment to go with the patterned one. If the individual needs additional help in knowing which things go together, code the clothing by putting color code dots on things that match.

3. Since all older adults do not live in congregate settings, Activities 1 and 2 can be carried out in the day program, but the clients' total wardrobe will not be available to use. Therefore, select a number of garments from your own wardrobe, or find some clothing similar to that worn by clients. Include some very basic work clothes, some sports attire, and some dress clothes. Some should be conservative and others patterned and brightly colored. Be sure to include some clashing colors and patterns. Use only pants or skirts, shirts, blouses, and tops. Begin with Activity 1, then go on to Activity 2.

4. Cut out of advertisements or catalogues pictures of these basic garments in a number of colors and patterns. Glue them to cards. Separate pants/skirts from blouses/shirts/tops. Have the clients match those that go together and identify those that clash.

Variations

1. Let each person select some garments and add to his/her present wardrobe from a catalogue.
2. Go to a shopping mall and observe how certain colors are emphasized each season. Decide which colors are "in" this year (season).

Materials

1. Basic items of clothing (pants, skirts, blouses, shirts, tops) in a variety of colors and patterns
2. Catalogues and color advertisements for clothing

Lesson B: Dressing for Special Occasions _____

Objectives

1. To be able to relate the kind of clothing worn to the occasion
2. To know what is appropriate in selected settings: work, home, sport, church, or party

Activities

1. From the previous lesson (Activity 4), there should be cards with pictures of basic items of clothing in a variety of colors and patterns. Add to these some pictures that clients cut out of catalogues and advertisements that show outfits suitable for dress-up occasions: suits, dresses, pantsuits, slacks, and shirts. Also add some active sports outfits.

   Label five shoe boxes: Work, Sport, Home, Church, Party. Scramble the cards and have each person take a turn sorting them.
2. Add some dress outfits to the collection of pants/tops gathered for the previous lesson. Have one person name an occasion and another respond by selecting the type of outfit appropriate to wear there.
3. Each person can start a scrapbook of choices of clothing using magazines, pattern books, and so forth.

Variations

1. Using the magazines, catalogues, and so on, decide "What would be a good outfit to wear to church; a restaurant; the park; a picnic; a party?"
2. Review or talk about accessories: jewelry, earrings, ties, etc.

Materials

1. Pictures of pants, skirts, shirts, and blouses from the previous lesson, plus more pictures and cards to add dresses, suits, and sports attire
2. Magazines, catalogues, and advertisements to cut out for scrapbook

Lesson C: Matching the Clothes to the Occasion

Objectives

1. To be able to select appropriate outfits for: work, sport, home, church, or party (church or party = dress-up)
2. To know which occasions demand special attention to dress

Activities

1. Use materials from Lessons A and B, which include lists of client's own wardrobe coded as to functional use and color coordination, pictures cut out and mounted showing appropriate clothing for various activities, and examples of well-matched outfits for each type of use (work, home, sport, church, party).

    Have each person use one of the sources of dress style to show what should be worn for these occasions:
    a. A picnic in the public park
    b. Going to a carnival
    c. Mowing the lawn
    d. Attending a church service
    e. Going to a dance at the workshop
    f. Going to exercise class
    g. Going to a nutrition site for lunch
    h. Going to a concert at the high school
    i. Playing miniature golf
    j. Going shopping at the mall

2. Videotape individuals dressed for different occasions. Keep them on camera for at least half a minute, walking and turning like models.

    Play back the tape and have the group name as many occasions as possible where that kind of outfit could be worn appropriately.

3. List all the places that members of the group have gone in the past couple of years, and either have them select pictures of the appropriate clothing for each or make a chart using the mounted pictures of various types of dress.

4. Do the same thing for places the members of the group are hoping or expecting to go in the future.

Variations

1. Have the clients cut pictures from magazines or newspapers showing a number of people at an activity such as picnic, family meal, party, sport event, restaurant. Discuss what is being worn by each participant in the activity.

2. When attending an activity with the group, call attention to the dress of other participants. Have them find those who are most appropriately dressed.

Materials

1. From previous activities: lists of each client's wardrobe, coded; pictures cut and mounted showing appropriate male and female attire for work, home, sport, church, party
2. Magazines to cut out pictures of group activities
3. Video camera, tape player

Unit IV. Taking Care of Clothing

Lesson D: Taking Care of Clothes _____

Objectives

1. To be able to hang up clothing on coat hangers
2. To be able to fold underwear, socks, tops, and sweaters, and place them in drawers neatly

Activities

1. Demonstrate the correct way to hang on hangers: coat, jacket, dress, pants, suit, rain-coat. (It is assumed that clients already know how to use hooks, since these are provided most often.)
2. Give each person a chance to practice with a partner who will tell when the task is done correctly so that the garment will keep its shape and wrinkles will fall out.
3. Demonstrate folding underwear: for ladies—underpants, slips, bras, stockings, socks; for men—shorts or briefs, t-shirts and underwear shirts, socks.
4. Provide a drawer (or drawer-shaped box) for each pair. Have same-sex pairs work to-gether to fold garments and place them in an organized way into the drawers so that a section of the drawer is used for each type of garment.
    • Discuss the advantage of having drawers neat and organized, so that one can tell how many of each type of garment remains, and when washing must be done to assure supply. Discuss how neatness is a trait that can be seen in the way each person stores possessions.
5. Demonstrate folding various kinds of sweaters: cardigans, vests, pullovers. Show how to smooth them and fold arms to prevent wrinkles. Let each person practice folding each kind.
6. Repeat the folding/putting in drawer activity using sweaters instead of underwear.

Variations

1. At the residence, have a drawer inspection and cleanup once a week, giving a special reward to those who pass inspection.
2. Appoint people to monitor how the coats are hung up at the day program or residence. (Be sure that hangers are available.)

Materials

1. Enough hangers for each person's use: shirt hangers, both clamp and clip hangers for skirts/pants, suit hangers (combination coat/pant hangers), coat hangers
2. Dresser drawer or box of that size for each pair of clients
3. Underwear, stockings, socks, tops, and other garments that are folded and stored in drawers; sweaters of several styles

Lesson E: Taking Care of Accessories and Shoes _____

Objective

1.   To know how to take care of accessories and shoes

Activities

1.   Display accessories that most people would have: scarves, gloves, ties, jewelry, hats. Ask people to tell which of these kinds of accessories they have.
     • Where do clients keep accessories when not in use: bedroom drawer, bathroom, cabinet, on special rack? Discuss the importance of keeping them in a place where they won't get messed up. Hang ties and scarves on rack or special hanger. Have a box for gloves; keep jewelry in jewelry box.
2.   Care of shoes
     a.   Canvas shoes can be washed in washing machine.
     b.   Running shoes should be wiped clean with damp cloth or sponge.
     c.   Leather shoes should be waxed and polished.
     d.   Leather boots can be treated with waterproofing or mink oil.
     • When leather shoes are not being worn, they should be on shoe trees. Demonstrate how to put in the trees, noting that they help the shoes go back to their original shape and thus they will look good and feel good longer.
     • Examine shoes for run-down heels and worn soles. Talk about taking shoes to shoe repair shop for new heels and soles.
3.   Demonstrate how to shine shoes and then let each person do it.

Variations

1.   Cut out pictures of shoes from advertisements and make a chart of types of shoes for men and women: work, sport, hiking, dress-up.
2.   Visit a shoe store or invite the manager of one to visit the group in order to find out what is recommended for shoe care.

Materials

1.   Shoes of all types: canvas, running shoes, sandals, leather dress shoes, boots
2.   Shoe care products: waxes, polishes, liquid shiners, brushes, buffers

Lesson F: Deciding About Cleanliness _____

Objectives

1. To be able to decide when a garment needs to be laundered
2. To know when a garment needs to be sent to the cleaners
3. To be able to use prewash spot removers for synthetics

Activities

1. Ask the clients how they decide when their clothes need to be laundered. Discuss:
   a. Which ones should automatically be put into the laundry hamper? (underwear, socks, t-shirts)
   b. Which ones might go through several wearings? (blouses or shirts, pants, cotton tops, sweat shirts)
   c. Which can be worn over and over until they need to be cleaned or laundered? (coats, jackets, sweaters)

   If clients need more than verbal instructions, use garments of each type and have three boxes there to place each garment in, making sure each person knows one box is for "washing after every wearing," one means "washing after several wearings," and the third box means "needs to be cleaned only when dirty."

2. Using clothing that has some spots and stains and even odor, discuss the signs that tell you that it's time to clean that garment. You may even want to point out missing buttons or zippers that have come unstitched.

   • Discuss how people feel about others who are dressed in messy, dirty, or smelly clothing. (They avoid that person and they almost never tell them why.)

3. Have each person inspect his/her own garments to look for wrinkles, dirt, stains, loose or missing buttons, detached zippers. Decide which garments need to be washed or cleaned, or need repair.

4. When stains are found on polyester or other synthetics, use prewash sprays or soaks on each spot, let it set for a minute, and then wash it out. Show how to do this on laundry day.

5. Set up a daily reward system for coming to program wearing neat, clean clothing. Have a Daily Dude Award . . . or Mr. or Ms. Clean. Put up photos of the people who win the awards. Be sure everyone knows who got the awards.

Variations

1. Visit a dry cleaner's shop to see how they operate; or go to a coin-operated laundry to do some washing. This is a step toward independent living.
2. Learn how to sew on buttons and stitch zippers down. It doesn't take that much talent to do these simple repairs; consider working on hems and pockets that are torn loose.

Materials

1. Garments with various kinds of soiling, wrinkling, stains, missing or loose buttons and zippers
2. Prewash spot removers and synthetic fabrics with spots or stains

SOCIAL INTERACTION (COMMUNICATION)

Unit V.   Conversation

Lesson A: Making Small Talk _____

Objectives

1.   To be able to talk to another person using ordinary small-talk topics and responses
2.   To distinguish between acceptable and unacceptable topics for conversation with strangers/acquaintances

Activities

1.   Model an interaction between acquaintances in which conventional small talk is the only conversation. Have two staff persons role play meeting in the morning before work starts and asking how each feels (did they have a good weekend, how does the weather look/feel); conclude with something like, "Have a good day."
2.   Pair up the group and have them practice the same kind of dialogue to do before the group. The topics may only be weather, how do you feel, did you have a good day or evening, and maybe, how is the family. Present the small-talk greetings and applaud those who do it convincingly.
3.   Discuss why there is small talk. Discuss the ideas that underlie the widespread use of small talk.
     a.   It's like a game everyone knows how to play and no one wins or loses. It's a non-threatening way of expressing interest in others.
     b.   It expresses good will toward others without being personal. If you want to talk more to the person, you can go from that, but if you don't want to, just say the expected and leave.

Role Plays for Staff or Clients

1.   Molly has a bad headache because she was up all night with an upset stomach from eating too much junk food and drinking too much at a party that night. She meets Joan, who was at the party, but whom she doesn't know.
     a.   She tells Joan all about her headache and upset stomach, and Joan obviously isn't interested and only wants to get away from her.
     b.   When Joan asks her how she is, Molly says, "Fine." When Joan asks if she had a good evening, Molly says, "Yes, it was a good party."
     Which way was better for making Joan like Molly? Which made Joan only want to get away from Molly?
2.   (In this dialogue one person tries to keep it impersonal and the other keeps asking very personal questions.)
     Joe is introduced to Bill and puts his hand out to shake. Bill shakes his hand and sees a ring on the finger, asks where he got the ring, how much did it cost, is it his wedding ring, is he divorced, how many children does he have, how much money does he earn, and so on. Joe avoids answering, tries to change the subject, but Bill just keeps on asking personal questions. Finally Joe just excuses himself and walks away.
     How did Joe feel about being asked personal questions? Was the information any of Bill's business? What did Joe say to let Bill know he didn't want to answer?

Variations

1. Ask each person to be a listener and reporter. They are to try to hear small-talk conversations and remember them to tell the group about.
2. Watch TV and see if small talk appears on any of the shows or movies; report on what is observed.

Materials

1. Papers or cards with the role plays written on them

Lesson B: What to Talk About _____

Objectives

1.　To know how to talk to others about topics that will be interesting and not annoying
2.　To be able to decide whether a topic is acceptable or not

Activities

1.　Some topics are "safe" to talk to almost anyone about. First try to get the clients to name some, then give hints. As topics are suggested, list them under *Good* or *Not Good*. Some that might be suggested are: weather, sports, cars, hobbies, movies, TV shows, food, diets, what happened in the news, health problems, feelings about others, personal information, religious beliefs, politics, who loves whom, something awful someone said about someone else, and so forth.

2.　Divide into pairs and practice talking about good topics. Staff may need to keep ideas flowing. People may take turns talking with staff, who will respond but will not bring up topics unless the other person is at a loss to think of something to say.

3.　Record in advance on videotape (or audiotape) some conversations that appear in television shows. After each topic is introduced, stop the tape and discuss whether that is a good thing to talk about to people you don't know too well. It may be necessary to have staff role play in advance to get the tapes.

4.　Videotape or record a news program, then present it item by item to the group so that they can decide what might be said in conversation about that event.

Variations

1.　Cut out pictures of newsmakers and events from weekly news magazines. Make a bulletin board showing ideas for conversation. Practice using the topics.

2.　Make cards with "good" and "not good" topics portrayed, such as are listed above. Have people take turns talking about the topics that are acceptable, and ignoring those that are not.

Materials

1.　News magazines: *Time, Newsweek,* and so forth
2.　Scissors, glue, and mounting for pictures

Lesson C: Meeting New People

Objectives

1. To know how to make simple introductions
2. To know how to respond to introductions

Activities

1. Staff models how to make a simple introduction. Give the names and a brief idea of who the people are. For example, "This is Bill; he came to visit today." The clients should carry on a small-talk-type conversation. ("I am glad you came to see us"; "How do you like what you have seen"; "I hope you will enjoy your visit.")
2. Discuss how the introduction should be done. Emphasize saying the name loudly and clearly, and if possible saying a little something to get the conversation going. Talk about shaking hands.

   • Discuss how the small talk helps people feel comfortable with each other because they both know what they are expected to say. Talk about expected responses and practice them: How are you? I'm happy to meet you; It's good to be here; This is a nice place; I enjoy being here; Is this your first time here? and so forth.
3. Tape record or videotape clients introducing each other to a staff person. Review the tapes to see whether the names were distinct and the people were able to help each other feel comfortable.
4. Practice shaking hands with firm grips. Often this is needed because the person with developmental disabilities offers a "dead fish" hand.

Variations

1. *Role Play:*   There is a party at the workshop. You see a person of the opposite sex you'd like to talk to and get to know. Introduce yourself and start a conversation that will attract the other person to you.
2. *Role Play:*   You are a visitor at a senior center; you are introduced to a person about your age and same sex. Keep a conversation going for one minute after you are introduced.

Materials

1. Video or audio recorder

Unit VI. Behavior in Public

Lesson D: Knowing What to Expect _____

Objectives

1. To be able to talk about apprehensions concerning going to a new place
2. To identify information needed for going somewhere new
3. To know how to go about getting that information

Activities

1. Form a small group circle, a sign that you are going to discuss feelings and talk about how to deal with situations. Ask clients if they can remember how they felt when they went somewhere new and strange for the first time: uneasy, scared, shy, withdrawn.
   a. Share with them that everyone feels these feelings when they go somewhere they haven't been, especially if it is very different from what they are used to. Give an example from your own experience of going to a strange place where you didn't know what to expect.
   b. Invite them to share their own experiences.
   c. Ask them to think about how they felt after they had been there for a while. It may be that they remember leaving an institution for a group home, or entering the workshop program. Talk about what helped them to get over the strangeness: making friends, staff helping them feel at home, learning what was expected of them and knowing they could do it.
   d. Tell from your own experience how you got over feeling strange, who helped you, how you found out what was expected of you and realized you could do it.
   e. Have group members share their own experiences.
   f. On a chart list in one or two words the ideas discussed; even those who can't read the words may remember these for as long as they are being presented. Keep the chart for future use.

2. Talk about how people find out what they can expect in new places and groups, using small group discussion as above.
   a. They talk to others who have been there.
   b. They send someone to find out.
   c. They ask someone who works there.
   d. They phone and ask for information.
   • If this group wants to go somewhere they don't know much about, how will they get the information they need about what is expected of them?
   a. Send someone from staff to visit the place and come back and tell everyone about it.
   b. Have someone from staff telephone the place for information.
   c. Invite someone from the new place to come talk to the group.
   List these on the chart and keep for use when actually planning to go somewhere new.

3. What kinds of information do we need about new places we want to go? Using small group discussion as above, ask the group for ideas that can be put on the chart and discussed. Keep these ideas or modify them. After all the ideas have been given, suggest those not mentioned.
   a. What do they do at this place?
   b. How much does it cost to get in—or how much should we plan to spend there?

    c.   What kinds of people go there?

    d.   What kinds of clothes are worn there?

    e.   Do we need to take our own food?

    f.   Where do we put our coats, boots, and so forth?

    g.   Do they have ramps and special toilets for handicapped people?

    h.   Do we have to know how to do anything special (set tables, play games) in order to take part?

Variations

1.   Reverse the situation and talk about what a new person coming to the workshop would need to know, and what present clients could do to make that person feel less scared.

2.   Work out the answers to the questions in Activity 3 above using the workshop or group home as the "new" place.

Materials

1.   Chalkboard, chart paper, marking pens

Lesson E: Going by the Rules _____

Objectives

1. To realize that every setting has its conventions and rules
2. To know how to find out what the rules and conventions are in the new setting

Activities

1. Give each pair of clients a board game to play. Tell them that they don't have to follow the rules, each player can just do what he wants to do. The only thing is that they must take turns and change every 30 seconds. After a few minutes, stop the games. Discuss:
   a. Was it more fun to play without rules?
   b. Did you enjoy it when the other person did whatever he/she wanted?
   c. Did it seem fair?
2. Every place has rules. On a chart list the rules of the workshop as people say them. Some are written down or on charts; others are just common knowledge. Find charts if they are on the walls somewhere.
   Discuss the reason for each rule. For example:
   a. Don't talk when you're supposed to be working. (You not only keep yourself from working and earning money, but you keep others from it also.)
   b. Put tools in proper place when not using them. (You can find them when you need them; people don't get hurt; tools don't get broken.)
   • Are there rules that need to be made so that this group would run better? Talk about it. Are there ways of acting that we don't have written rules about, but everyone knows that's the way you are supposed to act? (no stealing, hitting, pushing, shouting, etc.)
3. Discuss behaviors and rules in other places and some places where people behave in special ways. Discuss and act out the special ways people act in these places: football game, concert, church, restaurant.

Variations

1. Make a rule chart for the room and illustrate it with pictures from magazines.
2. Go to a restaurant, concert, or some special place with the idea of having everyone watch how others act so that it can be discussed by the whole group after the outing.

Materials

1. Chart paper, marking pen, magazines

Lesson F: Expressing Approval and Disapproval _____

Objectives

1. To be able to express approval and disapproval in socially acceptable ways
2. To know that approval and disapproval are expressed according to the setting
3. To increase the repertoire of social behaviors

Activities

1. Show videotape of children expressing excitement—jumping, shouting, waving their arms. Stop the tape and discuss how children show their approval (liking).

    Show videotape of people at a ball game, screaming, yelling, jumping. Stop the tape and discuss how everyone can show their excitement and support for a team at a sport event, and that kind of behavior is okay.

    Show videotape of an audience applauding after a concert. Stop the tape and discuss; this is how people show approval in a theater.

    • Children and adults express excitement and approval/disapproval differently. It is best for adults to act like adults.

    Approval and disapproval are expressed differently in different places. It is best to do as others do.

2. *Sociodramas*

    • At the Special Olympics your best friend is running in the 50-yard dash. It looks like someone else is going to win, but your friend pulls out ahead and takes first place. Show how happy that makes you.

    • Three of you set up seats like a theater. Sit down and listen to a lady playing the piano at a concert. When she finishes, show that you like it.

3. Videotape the sociodramas when you get them the way you want. Show them to the group and to others in the workshop.

Variations

1. Go to a sports event with the idea of watching others to see how many different ways people show excitement. Does everyone shout and jump around? Are some people quiet?
2. Reverse the sociodramas above. Have those attending the football game clap politely when the team scores, and those attending the concert scream and jump up and down after the pianist finishes playing.

Materials

1. Videotape, camera, player

Lesson G: The Right Way of Touching

Objectives

1.   To be able to express affection appropriately
2.   To know socially acceptable ways of touching others

Activities

1.   *Be sure you really know your clients and how they react to being touched before you do this activity.* If they can tolerate being touched, form a small group. Go to each one and hold hands for about half a minute as you look into their eyes. Discuss how that made each of you feel; what does it mean to hold someone's hand longer than to shake it? When people like each other, do they hold hands sometimes?
2.   Repeat the exercise above doing these things to each:
     a.   Put one arm around their shoulder
     b.   Hug them for a couple of seconds
     c.   Touch their upper arm
     d.   Touch their face or hair

     What message does each touch give to the person touched? Does it bother anyone to be touched by the leader? (It's okay to feel that way.) Who can touch us in these ways without making us feel uneasy? How would we feel if someone we didn't know touched us in these ways?

     What are some places we should not touch or be touched except by lovers or doctors?
3.   The only place you can touch someone you don't know well is on the hands—shaking their hand when you meet. Everything else is only for someone you know very well, well enough to know that it's okay to touch.
4.   *Sociodramas*
     • A new person comes to the workshop for the first day. Introduce her to the other members of the group. Everyone shakes her hand except one person, who tries to hug her. She is scared.
     • Your best friend came to the workshop today feeling very sad because her dog died. She starts to think about it while she works, and begins to cry. Comfort her.
     • Two of you go to a senior center nutrition site to have lunch with the other senior citizens. One of the senior citizens introduces himself to you and your friend. Shake hands.
     • Joan just got a new permanent, the kind that is very curly. You wonder how that hair feels with all the tiny curls. How do you find out?

Variations

1.   Discuss what to do when someone touches you in the places no one should. What should you do at the time, and who should you tell afterward?
2.   How can you let people know that you don't like to be touched? List all the ways you can think of and act them out.

Materials

1.   No materials needed unless you want to videotape the sociodramas

PERSONAL SECURITY (DAILY LIVING)

Unit VII.   Personal Information

Lesson A: What Personal Information Is Needed _____

Objective

1.   To know what personal information is needed by others

Activities

1.   *Role Play:*   You are a person who has just come into the workshop. The group must find out all about you so that you can take part. Let them ask questions, and ask why it is important to know that information.

   What is your name? Where do you live? Do you work somewhere? What is your phone number? Who will be home to answer?

   Write the information asked for on the board. Discuss. This information will be needed by anyone trying to enroll you or to help you.

2.   Use the list below and have the clients think of as many examples as they can of how the information is used.

   a.   Name: to know what to call you; to know how your name is spelled; to know how it should be on official papers and checks.

   b.   Address: to know where you live; where to send letters to you or your family; to decide which bus route you are on.

   c.   Phone number: to be able to phone you or your family; to know where to call if you are ill; to call you if the workshop is closed or plans are changed at the last minute.

   d.   Social Security number: so that you can be paid properly and records kept— because there is only one person in the United States with that number, but many people may have the same name; so they can be sure you are the right person with that name.

   e.   Age: to prove that you are the right age to get services from senior centers, nutritional sites, and so forth.

Variation

1.   Get some application forms and look at the kinds of information required to get licenses, library cards, bank accounts, and other services

Materials

1.   Application forms

Lesson B: Communicating Personal Information to Others _____

Objective

1. To know how to convey personal information to others

Activities

1. Make a transparency of a mock-up identification card similar to the one used in the workshop. Leave the spaces blank until someone from the group volunteers to be the person to get the ID card. Fill in the information with the assistance of the volunteers and the use of permanent records.
2. Be sure that each person has an ID card that has up-to-date information. Use the cards in these role plays:
    a. You are applying for a job at a local garden center. The manager asks how to spell your name.
    b. You have moved and want to be sure that the church secretary knows where to mail the church newsletter.
    c. You met a new friend at the senior center; you want that person to call you when he will be going to lunch again at the center.
    d. *(Pick someone with a fairly common name.)* You won a prize at the county fair drawing and someone else with the same name is trying to collect.
    e. You are going to lunch at a senior citizens' nutrition program. They ask you to prove that you are over age 60.

Variations

1. Get together several driver's licenses from staff. Let each pair of clients find the different information items on the license.
2. Talk about the uses of driver's licenses for identification (e.g., check cashing).

Materials

1. Transparency of mock-up identification card, marking pen
2. Identification cards for each person; several driver's licenses

Unit VIII.   What to Do When Help Is Needed

Lesson C: When Do You Need Help? _____

Objectives

1.   To be able to recognize situations in which help is needed
2.   To know who to ask for help

Activities

1.   Read or tell these stories, then ask what help was needed. Where would you get help?

   a.   Bill and Joe went by themselves to see the Cleveland Indians play baseball. They had been with their group several times and they knew how to ride the buses. They even had a copy of the bus schedule so they wouldn't have any trouble getting home. When they got ready to leave, Bill couldn't find his good jacket. They went to the Lost and Found, where the man told them that the sweepers would turn in anything they found after the stadium was swept. By the time they got the jacket the last bus had left and they were stuck at the stadium. What should they do? Who could they phone?

   b.   Helen and Ruth went shopping in a grocery store in their neighborhood. While they were walking around, Ruth got dizzy and sick. Helen found her a chair, then went to look for help. Who should she look for? What phone calls might she ask them to make?

   c.   Walter got ready to go to lunch in the workshop and he couldn't find his wallet. He had it on break because he bought a coke with some of his own money. He was afraid someone might have taken it on purpose, or maybe he lost it. Who should he tell about it? What should he say?

   d.   Loraine was at the movies with a friend when she went to the restroom. There, someone had dropped a lit match into a wastebasket and the paper towels had caught on fire. What should Loraine do?

Variations

1.   (*Group members*) Tell about a time when you were in an emergency situation and how you acted. Did anyone help? How did it turn out?
2.   (*Leader*) Tell about situations in which help was given and disaster prevented, and in which help was not given and disaster happened.

Materials

1.   None

Lesson D: Telephoning for Help or Information ——————————————

Objectives

1. To be able to use a phone to summon assistance
2. To be able to use a phone to get information

Activities

1. Get two discarded telephones from the phone store. Place one on a small table with a message pad and pencil available. Let clients use that phone to make emergency calls. The other phone should be answered by staff using these role plays:

    a. You are at church and everyone except the pastor has gone home. No one from the group home has come to pick you up. Call home.

    b. You are at the grocery store getting food for a party at the workshop. You got the soda pop and potato chips, but you forgot what else you were supposed to buy.

    c. You are at home when the phone rings and someone asks if Joan is there. You say, "Sorry, she is out now." They leave a number for her to call back when she comes in.

    d. You want to use senior transportation to go to an activity at the senior center. Call "Information" (Directory Assistance) for the number, and then call to see if you can be picked up at 11:00 on Tuesday to go to Golden Age Center.

    e. You are at home when someone calls and tells you that the party at the workshop will be on Friday at 7:00 and you are to tell everyone at your group home when it will be.

2. Give each person a card to list special telephone emergency numbers. They will want numbers for home, workshop, doctor, dentist, friend, police, and fire. Laminate the cards.

Variations

1. Let group members take turns making real phone calls to the workshop or group home to ask for information agreed on in advance.

2. (*Leader*) Act as a person who is making a call at the request of an older adult who needs help. Older adult needs to give the phone number and the message to the person making the call.

Materials

1. Two discarded telephones, note pad, pencil
2. Telephone directory or list of numbers
3. Cards for emergency numbers (to be laminated)

COMMUNITY ACTIVITIES (DAILY LIVING)

Unit IX.   Geography of the Community

Lesson A: Knowing Where Things Are _____

Objectives

1. To be able to locate areas of the community (to be determined in each locality) or to be aware of what is meant by them
2. When in a given area, to be able to identify it to others; for example, downtown, at the mall, residential area, park, fairgrounds, and so forth

Activities

1. Try using a map of the area for those clients who might be able to master the concept. Let the others just watch so that they get whatever they can of the concept.

    Tell them what the map shows: (this is the _____ city or _____ county.) Use highlighters to show the areas that you want them to learn: downtown, the mall, the park, the sports field, residential areas (where most houses are).
2. Show pictures or slides of the various areas and put them on the map with tape loops. Relate the areas to the kinds of use to which they are put:

Area	Use
Downtown	Stores, offices, banks, restaurants
Mall	Stores, banks, travel agencies, exhibits, restaurants, grocery stores
Park	Grass, flowers, paths, picnic tables, baseball diamonds, swim pool, swings
Residential	Houses, apartments, some offices, small shops, some gas stations

3. Find pictures in magazines that show the different uses of areas and make a montage for each type of area.
4. Take a van ride around to see the different areas. Have each person name the area and tell what can be seen that indicates the use of the area.

Variations

1. Make a scrapbook of photos of the various areas showing the uses to which they are put.
2. Put the map flat on a table. Make a schematic map–like representation on large paper showing the relative positions of the various areas. Color them differently.

Materials

1. Map of the city or county
2. Photos of various areas of the city or county
3. Magazines with pictures of types of areas to make montage
4. Construction paper or newsprint to make tabletop map

Lesson B: Knowing Where the Interesting Places Are ————————————

Objectives

1. To know what interesting places are in the community
2. To have a general idea where these places are located

Activities

1. (This activity is just to familiarize the clients with some of the places in the community where they go or might be interested in going. It is not important that they develop map skills. This is just an age-appropriate way of introducing the topic.)
   Ask the people to think of all the places they have been in the community:
   a. For outings to restaurants, parks, shows, and so forth.
   b. For shopping for food, clothing, TVs, stereos, and so forth.
   c. For entertainment—movies, sport events, exhibits, and so forth.
   List these on chalkboard or chart to use in the next activity.
2. On either the wall map or the tabletop map from Lesson A, mark the major points of interest with toothpick flags. They can be set in bits of clay for the tabletop map. Color code the categories: outings, shopping, entertainment.
3. Make a good chart showing the major points of interest in categories. Get a photo to illustrate each (or a picture cut from a magazine). Keep it, and as time passes and you visit the places, add photos of members of the group enjoying the places.

Variations

1. Ask the managers or representatives of some of the points of interest to come make a presentation to the group about what there is to do at these places.
2. Take a trip in the van to visit all the places in a category, for example, the restaurants or the movie houses. If someone has a camera, take pictures for the wall chart.

Materials

1. The maps from the previous activity, wall-size and tabletop
2. Toothpicks and paper to make location flags
3. Photos of places of interest in the community

Unit X. Available Services and Activities

Lesson C: Senior Citizen Activities in the Community _____

Objectives

1. To be aware that there are special activities in the community for senior citizens
2. To become interested in participating in senior activities

Activities

1. Invite a nonretarded older adult who is active in senior activities in the community to come talk about what is available for older adults. Ask that person to bring slides, if possible.
2. Send out explorers from the group (with escorts) to visit senior centers or nutrition sites, or to go to an activity. Ask them to tell what it was like.
3. Collect newspaper clippings about activities of seniors in the community—parties, trips, information on nutrition sites. Read these into a tape recorder and have the group listen to the tape and stop it when one is finished. Discuss each item. Display the clippings.

Variations

1. Send a staff person to a senior activity site and have that person report back, bringing tape recordings and photos
2. Take a small group, not more than three or four, to a senior nutrition site for lunch. Have them discuss how they enjoyed it or what they felt needed to be improved.

Materials

1. Newspaper clippings about senior citizen activities

Lesson D: Locating Places to Shop in the Community —————————

Objective

1. To be able to select and locate places in the community to shop for clothing, furnishings, supplies, and groceries

Activities

1. Ask the group to list all the things they go to stores to buy. List them on a chart as they are suggested. Talk about the kind of stores where each can be purchased: department store, drug store, discount store, grocery store. Choose a symbol for each type of store and place it before each item on the list.
2. Go for a drive or just remember the various kinds of stores in the community (limit it to those actually shopped in). Relate that list to the more general types in Activity 1 above.
3. Cut out advertisements for each of the stores in the community and make a display according to type. Ask each person to tell about something bought in one of the local stores.
4. Visit a mall and list all the kinds of stores that are in it.
5. Go in groups of two to visit each type of store and just look around. Notice the different sections and how each is identified. Notice the ends of aisles (the specials). Note how sale items are displayed. Report back to the whole group.

Variations

1. Invite a store manager to come talk about the store, what items they carry, where they can be found, what is best about that store.
2. Take one or two persons at a time into the stockroom of a store to see how the stock is kept before display.

Materials

1. Local newspaper advertisements for stores

Lesson E: Exhibits in the Community

Objectives

1. To be aware of exhibits in the community
2. To know what is exhibited and where exhibits are held

Activities

1. Collect materials about exhibits in the community for months before starting this activity. When beginning the activity, present them to the group to see if they have heard about any of them or have attended any.

   Give out the posters, brochures, advertisements, and handouts about the exhibits to individuals or pairs. Have them be ready to tell what was exhibited, and where and when the exhibit was held. If this is too difficult, the leader should assist each person.
2. Have the group attend an exhibit or arts and crafts show. Afterward, have group members tell what was seen and ask how he/she felt about it.
3. Make a calendar for the room on which exhibits and shows in the next few months can be listed. Post advertisements and brochures near the calendar.

Variations

1. Go to a museum and see permanent exhibits. Make a list of museums and permanent displays in the community or in large cities that can be reached.
2. Plan and set up an exhibit of group hobbies or productions resulting from various group activities (such as the photo gallery), and invite workshop employees to come see it.

Materials

1. Brochures, advertisements, posters, handouts from exhibits
2. Calendar on which exhibits can be listed

Unit XI.   Dining

Lesson F: Types of Restaurants _____

Objective

1. To know that there are several types of restaurants to which clients might go in the community

Activities

1. Go for a drive around the community with the aim of seeing several types of restaurants. Point out these: fast-food places, chain restaurants, locally owned and operated restaurants, ethnic food restaurants. Take photographs of the fronts of each. Get menus or have leader copy chart and prices for future use.
   • Over time, cut out advertisements for all of the community restaurants from the newspaper. If some offer coupons or are in a local discount book plan, get those too.
   • Have clients use these materials to make display showing the types of restaurants and the related advertising and money-saving offers.
2. Focus on one type of restaurant each day. On that day, display the chart about that type. Use the menus to discuss these characteristics of that type of site:
   a. What kind of meals are served?
   b. Is it inexpensive, moderate, or expensive?
   c. What kind of seating, tables, silverware, and so on are used?
   d. Do you get the food yourself or are there waiters/waitresses?
   e. Do they have the same menu all the time, or does it change every day?
   f. Do you pay when you get the food or after eating?
   g. Are you expected to tip?
   Chart the answers to use for future occasions when getting ready to eat out at a restaurant.
3. Plan a visit to each kind of restaurant. If possible, take only two or three clients at a time. Review the type of restaurant as well as the specific place before going. The next day after the outing, review the chart and discuss the experiences each person had.

Variations

1. Have a waiter or waitress come tell about the kind of restaurant where he/she works.
2. Visit a fast-food restaurant and watch workers prepare the food. Visit the kitchen of a more conventional restaurant and see how the food is prepared and what the server does.

Materials

1. Photos of restaurants in the community; advertisements for restaurants, menus, coupons or discount offers

Lesson G: Ordering a Meal

Objective

1. To be able to order a meal in each type of restaurant

Activities

1. Use menus from the community restaurants to discuss how to order a meal. If possible, staff should role play ordering, or a videotape can be made in advance. For a regular (non-fast-food) restaurant, these concepts need to be discussed (or see Activity 2):

    a. What is an appetizer? Must everyone order one? Does it cost extra? What kinds of appetizers might you expect to have available?

    b. What kinds of salad might come with a meal? What different kinds of dressings are offered? How do you get just a salad for the meal? How do you fill your plate at a salad bar?

    c. For the entree or main course of the meal, what are the different kinds of meats one might choose from? What does it mean when meat is fried; sauteed; roasted; broiled?

    d. What are the choices of potatoes (baked, french fried, home-fried, boiled)? What does each look like? How do the tastes differ? How is each one eaten?

    e. What kinds of vegetables might be served? How are they eaten?

    f. Desserts are offered after the meal. Must you get one? What are the choices? Do they cost extra?

2. (These activities can be done as a unit lasting several weeks.) Various foods can be brought in to be seen, tasted, and learned. Pictures of each kind of food can be cut from magazines like *Ladies' Home Journal* or *Woman's Day,* and charts of the various foods can be made to relate to menus. Chances are that the clients have eaten these foods many times without ever learning the names or styles of preparation (fried, roasted, baked), so that they may recognize the food, but need help in learning names.

Variations

1. Most clients have had a lot of experience eating at fast-food restaurants, but they may not know all the choices available. On a trip to a fast-food place, have each person order something different and have a taste test.

2. Get pictures of the various choices in fast-food places, and make a chart about each place.

Materials

1. Menus from each type of restaurant studied
2. Pictures of food from magazines
3. Samples of foods as each is studied
4. Chart paper and mounting paper to make charts

Lesson H: How to Act in a Restaurant _____

Objectives

1. To be able to blend into the crowd at a restaurant
2. To be able to order, eat, and pay the check

Activities

1. Take a trip to a fast-food restaurant in the community with the idea that each person will be watching the other customers unobtrusively. How do they:
    a. Wait in line?
    b. Give their order?
    c. Pay the bill?
    d. Get seasonings, mustard, ketchup, sauces, etc.?
    e. Fill their plate if there is a salad bar?
    f. Act while eating?
    g. Discard their trash?
    This ought to be an easy activity because clients will already know a great deal about it. Make a chart using either words, pictures, or sketches to show the answers to the questions.
2. Role play going to a fast-food restaurant going through all the steps above. Videotape and view the results. Decide how well it was carried out.
3. Go to a regular restaurant and observe these things unobtrusively:
    a. How do customers get seated? Do they sit where they want? Does someone take them to a table?
    b. How do the customers get the menu? Who takes the order? What do the customers do while waiting for their meal?
    c. What part of the meal comes first? How is it eaten? What do the customers do to show they are ready for the next part of the meal?
    d. How do they eat the main part of the meal? How do they show that they are finished? Do they clear any part of the table?
    e. Do they have dessert? Coffee with meal or after?
    f. Do they leave a tip? Where do they put it? How much should they leave?
    Return to the group and discuss what was seen. Role play the whole sequence a number of times until everyone has had a turn. Videotape the person who does it best, play the tape, and discuss the high points.
4. Compare the charts of the answers to the questions in Activities 1 and 3, and compare the customs of the two restaurant types, fast-food and conventional. Emphasize that the same people go to both kinds of places but they observe the customs of the place where they are, and that they learn what is expected of the customer by observing others. (For example, at McDonald's you are expected to put your trash in a container; at Wendy's you leave everything on the table.)

Variation

1. Videotape staff role playing going to either kind of restaurant and making some very obvious mistakes that call attention to themselves. (Don't get carried away and overdo it; you don't want to emphasize wrong behavior.) Have the group watch the film and point out mistakes.

Materials

1. Videotapes
2. Chart paper

PUBLIC TRANSPORTATION (Daily Living)

Unit XII.   Destination

Lesson A: Where Are You Going? _____

Objective

1. To be able to state or have written the address of a destination

Activities

1. Use the materials gathered for the community activities in the preceding section. Display the choices of places to which one might go in the community. Have each client select a place and identify where on the literature the address can be found. Evaluate clients' ability to say and remember the address. If it is reliable, have them write the address only for emergency use. If the person can't say or remember addresses, make him/her a card showing the name of the event, place, and address.
2. Have the group practice using the cards to show each other where they are going in the community.
3. Use the personal ID cards from Lesson B in Unit VII to identify the destination that one would give in returning from a community activity.

Variation

1. Make other cards for individuals with the addresses of relatives, friends, the workshop, church, or any other important place.

Materials

1. 3 × 5 cards to write addresses on
2. ID cards for each individual

Lesson B: How to Get There ————————————————————————

Objectives

1. To become familiar with bus routes in the community
2. To be able to decide whether to use bus or taxi to get to a destination

Activities

1. Get copies of the local bus schedule for each client. Contact the bus company to get a map of the bus routes. If it is not large enough for everyone to see, draw the routes in on a large area map using a different color felt marker or highlighter for each route.

    Put one route on at a time and spend time having those people who would use the route become familiar with where that bus goes.
2. Use the bus schedules to identify the times that the bus will be at the stop nearest either the residence or the workshop. Note how often the buses run and be sure the people who would use the route know that. If they can't remember, either write it on a card or draw on small clock faces to be kept in the wallet.
3. On the large map used in Activity 1, place red dots on community activity locations that might be visited and label them. Spend a day at least going over this information until the people feel secure about it. If they want to have addresses of destinations written down for future use, print them on a card. If reading is a problem, use symbols.
4. For destinations that are not near bus lines, suggest that a taxi will take the passenger right to the door of the destination. Place on the large map green dots to represent taxi-only destinations.

    Go over these and emphasize that these can be reached only by cars or taxi. Discuss situations in which there might not be a private car to take one.

Variations

1. Take individuals or pairs on a bus ride on the route they would use to go to community activities. Point out landmarks that will help them know where they are and whether they are near a stop for a destination.
2. Role play a situation where an individual needs to call a taxi, such as needing to go to one of the destinations where bus service is not available.

Materials

1. Bus schedules, route maps for bus lines
2. Felt markers or highlighters
3. Press-on dots—red and green

Unit XIII.   Using Buses

Lesson C: Catching the Right Bus

Objectives

1. To be able to find the nearest bus stop
2. To be able to identify the bus that should be hailed

Activities

1. Using the large area map from Activity 1 in Lesson B, put a circle around the bus stop nearest the workshop and then, for each client, the one nearest where he/she lives.

    Take the group to the stop nearest the workshop, pointing out the way as you go. When they get there, take a group photo at the site. Place the photo on the wall next to the map with an arrow pointing to the stop.
2. Take individuals to the stop nearest their residence and take photos of them waiting there. Put those photos on the wall next to the map with arrows pointing to the stop.
3. One at a time, make large cardboard signs with the information identifying each bus that would be used. Spend a whole period learning what the sign looks like, what the route number is, where that route goes, what community activity destinations are on that route, and where the bus stop is.
4. When all the relevant routes are learned, reinforce the learning by giving one person a destination card from the first activity in this section, and having that person select the card identifying the right bus and point on the map to the stop nearest either home or workshop to catch that bus.

Variations

1. Give each person a bus identification card and have them point out the nearest stop for that bus and one place in the community one might want to go on it.
2. Go to either the nearest stop or downtown where a number of routes pass and read the bus identifications with a small group. Relate each one to destinations.

Materials

1. Map from previous activity
2. Cards with bus identifications
3. Camera and film

Lesson D: Paying Bus Fare _____

Objective

1.   To be able to select the correct amount to pay bus fare

Activities

1.   Put on a table a small coin purse with about 5 quarters, 8 dimes, 5 nickels, and a dollar bill in it. Tell the group that this is their coin purse and that they will need to pay bus fare out of it. Have someone empty it on the table and arrange the coins by type.
     • Review the value of the coins and practice selecting requested coins.
2.   On a chart or chalkboard, write the amount of local bus fare. Ask which coins would be needed to make exactly that amount. When the simplest answer has been given, write the number and coin amounts on the chart (75 cents = 25 + 25 + 25; 75 cents = 3 quarters) or paste actual coins on the chart.
3.   For those who are able to do coin equivalents, practice making the amount using a variety of coins.
     • Don't include those who are not able to do coin equivalents. For them the safest thing is to know one way. Have that group make cards with cutouts of the coins and practice getting those coins together.

Variation

1.   Ride a bus and have each person select the correct fare and put it in the coin box.

Materials

1.   Coins: 5 quarters, 8 dimes, 5 nickels, and a dollar bill
2.   Coin purse
3.   3 × 5 cards
4.   Chart paper or chalkboard

Lesson E: Where to Get Off

Objective

1. To be able to get off the bus at the destination

Activities

1. Take a small group on a bus ride with the objective of having them watch how each person signals to get off. If possible, ask a passenger how the destination can be anticipated and what is done to signal, or just point out those landmarks that indicate that the destination is near.

2. For those who are not able to distinguish landmarks, suggest that they tell the driver their destination and then sit near the driver so that they will hear that destination announced.

3. *Role play (Use the destination cards from Lesson A in Unit XII):* Each person has a turn being the driver and being the passenger. Have the passenger get aboard, pay the fare, and tell the driver what destination is needed and ask for assistance. Driver acknowledges and then tells that person when to get off ("Next stop for _____").

Variation

1. Take a ride on a bus to a senior activity or a community activity; have the person give the destination and ask for assistance in getting off at the right stop.

Materials

1. Destination cards from previous activities

Unit XIV.   Taxis

Lesson F: Calling for a Taxi _____

Objective

1.   To be able to call for a taxi

Activities

1.   Cut out and mount on cardboard advertisements for local taxi services from old telephone directories.
2.   Look at each advertisement to see what it tells: name of company, address of company, phone number. Highlight the phone number.
3.   Discuss how taxis differ from buses:
     a.   They pick you up wherever you are.
     b.   They go right to the destination.
     c.   Up to three people can ride.
     d.   Passengers share the total fare.
     e.   Driver should be tipped.
4.   Using the phone and destination cards from Unit VIII, Lesson D and Unit XII, Lesson A, role play phoning the taxi service and telling your location and destination.

Variation

1.   Repeat the role play where an individual called for a taxi in a situation where bus services were not available (Variation 2, Lesson B, Unit XII). Call for the taxi and give the location where it should pick up and the destination.

Materials

1.   Telephones and destination cards

Lesson G: Paying Fare and Tipping ————————————————

Objectives

1. To be able to pay the right amount for taxi fare
2. To be able to tip

Activities

1. *Taxis that charge by zone:* Get a map of the zones with the charges for going to each. Go over it carefully with those clients who want to learn about zone charges. Practice figuring the fare between zones.
2. *Taxis that charge by meter:*
    Discuss the principle of meters—that the charge is based on distance traveled and that the only thing that matters to the passenger is the final amount shown on the meter.
    • Make a series of 3 × 5 cards showing different amounts as they would appear on the meter. Use the coin purse from the bus fare activity to make the fares with bill and coins. Have each person who wants to learn to use taxis practice this.
3. Tips should be 15%. This will be a challenge to teach. We suggest using either 10% or 20%. Figure 10% by taking the first two numbers of the fare and if it's not an even-nickel amount, going to the next higher nickel. For a real challenge, try to teach the concept of doubling the first two numbers and, if necessary, going to the next higher nickel!

    Or, Make a chart showing appropriate tips per dollar.

    Or, Tell clients to ask the driver because they can't figure how much it should be.

    Or, Tell clients to find out in advance approximately how much the fare will be for a particular trip and then to ask someone at the residence or workshop to figure out how much to tip.

Variation

1. Role play riding in a taxi, paying the fare, and tipping.

Materials

1. Information about zones and areas for taxis that use zones
2. Information about metered fares
3. 3 × 5 cards with metered fares on them
4. Coin purse with coins and bill from Lesson D, Unit XIII

LEISURE/RECREATIONAL ACTIVITIES

Unit XV.   Hobbies (Making Things)

Lesson A: Knitting and Crocheting _____

Objectives
1. To be aware of knitting and crocheting as possible hobbies
2. To be able to do at least one craft as independently as possible

Activities
1. Display a number of handmade articles that are knitted or crocheted or tatted. If possible, have the person who made the article talk to the group about how much it cost, how much time it took, what it will be used for, how that person learned to do the craft, and when time for it is found.
2. A number of well-written and illustrated how-to-do-it books can be found by the leader (no specific instructions for these crafts will be given here). Show the how-to-do-it book to the clients and explain how each picture illustrates a step in the process. Do a sample following the illustrations step by step. Then give the clients an opportunity to learn and practice the simplest stitches (knit and purl, single and double crochet, and tatting knots).
3. Make samples with the kinds of yarn or threads that will be used and measure each person's output for gauge. Write on a 3 × 5 card what the gauge is for that thread and size of needle for each person to keep.
   • Teach the knitter or crocheter to use a ruler to measure the length of what is being made.
4. Over time and after the learner is able to do the stitches with consistency, make a simple project, such as a scarf or granny square.
5. As they improve, teach clients to read patterns or have some simple standard patterns available for repetitious use (granny square, afghan strips, etc.). Encourage the person to work on the project when at home and bring it in for the leader to check out.

Variations
1. Make a permanent display of various sizes and colors of yarn and threads. Display the different needles and crochet hooks with samples of the size of stitch each one makes.
2. Use volunteers to help teach the craft, especially if they are willing to be continuing consultants to the individuals they teach.

Materials
1. Knitting needles and crochet hooks of all sizes
2. Various colors and sizes of yarn and crochet thread
3. Illustrated manuals teaching knitting and crocheting

Lesson B: Needle and Thread

Objective

1. To be able to make simple objects using hand sewing skills

Activities

1. Visit an arts and crafts exhibit where hand-sewn articles are displayed. Point them out to the clients. Ask one of the displayers to come tell about the craft and bring samples of handmade articles.
2. Ask the people to bring in personal items of clean clothing that need to be mended or have buttons sewn on. If the leader is not skilled in mending, invite someone who is able to do it. Have the articles mended with the group watching and hearing how it is done.
3. Teach clients to thread the needles:
   a. Cut a length of thread about 1 foot long.
   b. Moisten the thread end so that the strands stay together.
   c. Hold the needle so that the hole is facing you.
   d. Push the thread through and pull it out the other side.
   e. Make a rolled knot in the long end.
   f. Remember to always keep a long enough tail so that the needle doesn't come unthreaded.
   • Using cotton squares and needle and thread, teach clients to sew straight stitch, making the stitches as small as possible and following along a penciled line. Practice this until it is done well.
4. After a level of skill is attained, make a simple project. For example, get some stamped designs from a fabric store to make either small stuffed toys or stuffed Christmas ornaments. Cut them out, place right sides together, and stitch around using very small stitches and leaving an opening to stuff. Turn right-side-out and stuff with filling. Sew the opening with an overcast stitch (which must also be learned).

Variations

1. Learn to sew a hem, to sew on a button, to reseat a zipper, and to mend a torn armhole. Make a display for everyone to see of clothing that was mended by the owner. Give prizes for the best work.
2. At Christmas, decorate a tree with handmade stuffed ornaments and give the tree to a child or to the workshop or group home.
3. Make stuffed toys or ornaments to sell.

Materials

1. Cotton squares of material
2. Needles, thread
3. Yard goods printed with ornaments or animals to stuff
4. Polyester filling

Lesson C: Cooking

Objective

1. To be able to cook some specialties as a hobby

Activities

1. Take the group to a county fair to see the exhibit of baked goods. Talk to some of the exhibitors; invite one to talk to the group about the hobby of cooking and baking.
2. Discuss occasions when people need to take something they have made for everyone to share: picnics, family gatherings, church suppers, potlucks. If convenient, have a relative who likes to make special dishes for church suppers or potlucks come and talk about it.
3. Ask individuals to attend dinners at their churches and report to the group what was served and who made it. What was the most popular food? Did people ask for recipes? Would they like to invite members of the group next time?
4. Take a survey of the group to see what they would like most to be able to cook or bake. (It probably will be cookies, cakes, brownies, or pies.) Decide on one or two things to learn.
5. Go to a grocery store and see if the items chosen come in mixes or can be made as variants of mixes. Can pie filling be bought frozen or canned? Can pie crusts be bought frozen? Discuss the advantages of using prepared foods and adding to them to make them special.
6. Make the dishes as part of a group activity either at the program site or residence. The first time, just serve them to the group to see if they are satisfactory. When the skills are firm, make them for a special occasion or gift to someone.

Variations

1. Have a bake sale to earn enough money to buy more groceries in order to make special treats to take to someone who is ill or who has a birthday.
2. Inquire of the church that had the potluck dinner whether several of your group can come and bring along the specialty they learned to make.

Materials

1. Mixes and prepared foods for making cakes, pies, cookies, and so forth

Lesson D: Photography _____

Objectives

1. To be able to take pictures of people and places
2. To keep photos in a collection for a hobby

Activities

1. Go to a photography exhibit in the community. Have the clients pay particular attention to the content of the pictures and what makes each look special. How many are of scenery? How many are of people? Are the people just standing straight and looking at the camera or are they doing something interesting? Think of other features to observe and write them on a chalkboard or picture them in cartoon form as they are suggested.
2. Ask those who have them (including staff) to bring in photo albums and spend some time looking at the pictures to see how they differ from art photography. What features can be seen? Are the people easy to identify? Are they close enough to the camera? Is the light right? Are they just looking at the camera or are they doing something? Put these ideas on a chart too.
3. Have a person with a photography hobby bring equipment and some photos to the group. Pick someone who has relatively simple camera equipment (automatic focus and advance, for example), so that the people in the group will be able to follow that example if they choose this hobby.
4. The photography hobbyist can show each person how to pose people for pictures, how they should be placed, what kind of light is required and where it comes from, how far away the photographer should stand, and how to take a picture without moving the camera.
    • Give each person a chance to take a picture of the same person or small group. Have them also take a picture of a building or scene in the same way. Keep a record of who took each picture (by number). When the film is developed, decide who took good pictures and discuss what the differences in effect were.
5. Have each person bring in about 20 photos that need to be put in an album. Let each person purchase an album of the type that one just puts pictures in and smoothes a plastic cover over. Spend some time making pleasing arrangements of three to four photos on each page and then put them in the albums. If the effect is not pleasing, the photos can simply be removed and rearranged.

Variations

1. Bring in photos of the group activities that have accumulated over time and make an album for the enjoyment of everyone.
2. Take pictures of various aspects of the day or residential program and make an album to give to the director or superintendent for a gift.
3. Mount some photos in montage-style picture frames and hang them in the meeting room for a while before they are put in the bedroom of the person who took them.

Materials

1. Automatic-type camera for each participant
2. Film, photo album for each, montage-type picture frames
3. Photos that need to be put in albums

Lesson E: Woodworking

Objective

1. To be able to construct simple wood projects for a hobby

Activities

1. Either visit a craft display where woodcrafts are shown or find a person in the community who does woodworking and ask for a display before the group.
2. Visit in pairs or threes the woodshop at the local high school just after the students have left so that the instructor can talk about what they make and show the tools and machinery they use. Discuss what might be the simplest project to make and what skills are needed to do it.
3. Get samples of various woods from a local lumberyard. Make a display with labels and have those who are interested in this hobby learn what the different woods look like. Stain a piece of each kind of wood in its most usual stain.
4. Use the display of woods to identify the woods in various pieces of furniture. Note that some "woods" now are plastic formicas made to look like wood, but easier to clean and less likely to become damaged.
5. Use simple tools to learn and practice basic woodworking skills such as measuring, sawing, nailing, gluing, and sanding. Practice until each person is reasonably skilled at the basics.
6. Make a simple wood project following a diagram or pattern. Have a display of completed projects. Let each person describe what was made and the use to which it will be put.

Variations

1. Ask staff to bring in wood items that they have made and tell how they learned to do it, how much each item cost, and how it is used.
2. Go to a local gift shop or store and find out how much is charged for items made of wood.

Materials

1. Samples of various kinds of wood—some stained in usual color
2. Inexpensive pieces of wood and simple tools such as hammers, saws, nails, glue, sandpaper, screwdrivers, wood stains

Lesson F: Gardening

Objectives

1. To be aware of gardening as a hobby
2. To be able to select seeds or starter plants for a garden
3. To be able to prepare the ground for a garden
4. To be able to plant either seeds or small plants
5. To care for a garden—weeding, watering, spraying

Activities

1. In September, visit a backyard vegetable garden to see the produce on the plants. Harvest some tomatoes and whatever is easily prepared, such as beans or squash, and take them back to prepare and eat.
2. In late spring, visit a backyard garden to see how the soil is prepared and how seed or small plants are planted. Discuss every aspect of what is seen.
3. Visit the produce department of a supermarket and observe what fruits and vegetables are for sale. List those that could be grown in a backyard garden. Note the prices if that is important to the group.
4. Collect seed catalogues for vegetables and flowers and have enough so that some can be cut up and others used for reference. Use out-of-date catalogues to make charts showing the various vegetables that can grow in the area. Use the others for finding prices if seeds are to be mail-ordered.
5. Visit a seed rack in a store and look for seeds of plants that grow well in the area. List them or purchase a few packets for future use.
6. Select a plot for a garden at either the program site or the residence. Have the participants remove top growth, spade the garden, and if possible, add manure and work it in.
7. Decide what will be planted and where each variety will go. Decide whether to try to start with seed or buy starter plants. (Probably starter plants will be preferable to increase possible success.) Put in stakes and tie strings for straight lines for seed.
8. Find out how to test soil for moisture to determine if watering is needed. Find out about the need for additional fertilizer and set up responsibility for care. When weeds appear, show them to the group and be sure they can distinguish weeds from vegetables or flowers. When that is known, assign weeding duties.
9. Make a chart showing approximately when the fruits of the group's labors can be expected. Think about possible uses for the produce, such as: preparing them and serving them for lunch, freezing or canning, giving them to poor people, selling them, giving them as gifts.

Variations

1. Grow flowers to cut and put in vases for decorating the room or for giving to others.
2. Relate the garden activity to the study of the food groups; discuss what nutritional benefits come from eating vegetables fresh grown.

Materials

1. Seed catalogues, current and out-of-date
2. Charting paper or cardboard
3. A garden plot and tools for preparing it

Lesson G: Growing Houseplants
Objectives

1. To be aware of growing and caring for houseplants as a hobby
2. To recognize common houseplants
3. To be able to pot, water, fertilize, and start plants

Activities

1. Walk around the workshop and offices and notice the plants that people have for decoration. When you see someplace where there are a lot of plants, ask the owner what is liked about having plants around.
2. Visit a shop where houseplants are sold. Observe the various kinds of plants and look at the containers. See if the store has a catalogue or price list to give to the group.
3. Ask staff or relatives to contribute healthy examples of the common houseplants that could be left with the hobby study group for a month or so. If a houseplant hobbyist is available, invite that person to come talk to the group or even to act as a resource person for the time of the study.
4. Get books about houseplants: buy them if money is available, borrow if someone offers, or get them from the local library (ask for extended loan usually given to teachers). Look up the common plants and read about care. Do one plant a day. At the end, make a chart of general suggestions for plant care, either written or in sketch form.
5. Have a hobbyist or greenhouse operator demonstrate how to start plants from leaves or stems. Carefully cut starters from the donated plants and root them. When they are well rooted, demonstrate and practice potting them properly. (Instructions can be found in plant care books.)
6. If plants develop diseases or insect problems, consult the plant care books or a greenhouse operator for advice. Share it as much as possible with the participants.
7. Have a display of the plants grown from starters, then either give them as gifts or take them home.

Variations

1. Visit a greenhouse where houseplants are grown.
2. Learn to make or purchase macrame hangers and display some plants in hanging baskets.

Materials

1. Borrowed specimens of common houseplants
2. Pots, potting soil, sprays

Lesson H: Making a Scrapbook _____

Objective

1. To be able to collect and keep mementos of important events

Activities

1. Find someone who has kept a scrapbook and ask them to share it with the group. What was collected? Why were these things kept? How are they arranged and put into the scrapbook?

2. Discuss and list the important events in people's lives: births, weddings, baptisms, funerals, parties, dinners, graduations, anniversaries. Talk about the kinds of things one can save from these occasions: invitations, photos, programs, tickets, souvenirs. Bring in a number of things you have accumulated and intend to keep. Talk about how one could make a scrapbook to keep things in so they could be looked at again and again.

3. Get a scrapbook for each person who wants to make one. Clients can shop for one or you can buy them and sell them at cost. Have transparent tape, rubber cement, paste, and glue available. Let each person arrange mementos in some order and decide whether that is the best way to display them. Make a scrapbook.

4. When scrapbooks are finished, display them for everyone to see. Have each person in turn tell the whole group what the mementos are and what occasion they are reminders of.

Variations

1. Make a group scrapbook of souvenirs and pictures from events and parties done together.

2. Make specialty scrapbooks, such as a matchbook collection, stamps, photos of animals or sports stars, and so forth.

Materials

1. Scrapbooks—some already made, one new one for each person who wants to make one

2. Glue, transparent tape, rubber cement, scissors

3. Souvenirs, photos, mementos

Unit XVI. Amusements (Productive Use of Leisure)

Lesson A: Better Use of TV Time _____

Objectives

1. To be aware of television programs other than old favorites
2. To be able to select programs using a schedule

Activities

1. Ask each person to list favorite television shows; go around the group giving each one a chance until all favorites are listed on chart. Discuss why each is liked and list answers.
2. Provide a TV program guide for each person. Use highlighters to mark favorite programs in green. Look at the not-watched shows that conflict with favorites and decide why those are not ever tried.
    * Look at program descriptions to see what is on the unwatched shows; discuss how one who can't read could get the information about what is on the show that day. Discuss possibility that choices could be made instead of always watching same shows.
3. List these categories on the board or chart: talk show, game show, soap opera, crime/adventure series, comedy, nature, music, and any other that is appropriate. Classify the favorites and see if there is overviewing of a category.
4. Sample some rarely watched shows (in the residence) and discuss them. Are they interesting? Might they be worth watching from time to time? Are they educational? Might they stimulate new interest?
5. Use a yellow highlighter to identify new shows watched. Give them a rating from 1 to 10 (each viewer). Collect photos or cut out pictures of the performers in favorite shows and display them on the wall near the TV viewing chart. Continue over time to keep up the chart and change the photos.

Variations

1. It is harder to do this for radio because there is so little variety, but try to adapt some of the TV activities for radio listening.
2. Visit a TV or radio station in the area or go see local TV or radio personalities when they are broadcasting from a business or mall.

Materials

1. Local TV program guides for each person
2. TV fan magazines to cut up

Lesson B: Keeping a Pet

Objective

1. To be able to care for a pet

Activities

1. Have someone bring baby kittens or puppies to the group. Have someone else bring a bird, goldfish, gerbils, hamsters, guinea pigs, or other small pets. Give each person an opportunity to touch the creatures if he/she wants to. (We have found that many people who were in institutions are frightened of animals, so be sure the ones brought in are small and not threatening. Don't insist on everyone touching or petting them.) Spend some time just looking at them and enjoying their movements.
2. Make a display of pet pictures cut out of magazines. Mount the individual pictures or make a montage of dogs, cats, fish, birds, or other animals. (Many animals are rarely featured in advertisements, so you may have to use photos or sketches.)
3. Go to a pet store in a mall or to the pet department in a variety store and see what pets are for sale and how much each pet of interest costs. Place the locations where they can be bought and the prices on cards and tape them to the wall near the pictures of pets.
4. Bring in the classified advertisements for pets, especially from a Sunday paper. Read them to the group and talk about getting pets for free or inexpensively from noncommercial sellers or animal shelters.
5. Those who want to go farther into the subject can go to someone's home where an adult dog or cat can be visited. Discuss its care with the owner. Talk about how to pet, control, walk, and feed it, what medical care it needs, and where it sleeps. Ask questions.
6. For those who actually have or get a pet, visit a grocery store or buy and bring in various types of foods for the animal: dry, canned, semimoist, and snacks. Compare costs and convenience.
7. In a variety store, look at the various toys, bowls, beds, collars, chains, and accessories that may be needed to keep a pet properly. Discuss the costs and talk about the possibility of getting them from yard sales or other sources.

Variations

1. Ask someone from the local Humane Society to visit and discuss selection and care of small pets.
2. Bring a bowl of goldfish to the group and keep it in the room, giving everyone an opportunity to feed and change the water, if willing.
3. Get a parakeet and cage for the room and give everyone a chance to care for it.

Materials

1. Magazines with pictures of pets to cut out
2. If a store visit isn't possible, display of pet foods for those pets of interest

Lesson C: Playing Table Games _____

Objectives

1. To be able to play table games with other people
2. To be able to say which games one can play and which are not known

Activities

1. By the time people reach this age, they probably know how to play one game, or at least some members of the group can do so. Ask what games they can play. Have the boards and pieces available so that the games can be demonstrated for all to observe. Have those who know the games demonstrate them.
2. Pair each experienced player with someone who wants to learn the game. The leader first shows the way it is played; practice that, then give the rules as an occasion is encountered. Do not try to explain everything about the game before it is played—this kills motivation. Give daily time for practice. Don't keep scores or emphasize winning.
3. Rotate those who want to learn games through all the games over a period of weeks; do not change games in the middle of a day or week; be sure that one is mastered before another is tried, unless someone decides that a game is too difficult.
4. Teach a simple card game to a group of four people. UNO is good because there is little strategy involved. Fish requires memory and is often perceived as age-inappropriate for adults. Modified Rummy can be played requiring only three of a kind instead of runs to lay down. The important thing is that the game must be fun for the players.
5. Discuss the use of games in senior centers and day activity centers. Talking with partners or other players is a good way to have fun with others and get acquainted. Reinforce the idea that knowing how to play games is a good way to make new friends.

Variations

1. If people can tolerate competition, have a tournament in checkers or some other game most people know. Reward the winner of each round.
2. Ask other staff to play with group members in order to give practice in conversation and fun with others.

Materials

1. Table games such as checkers, Parcheesi, any other adult-style marker-mover game
2. Card games: UNO, rummy, and other adult-looking card games

Lesson D: Playing Active Games _____

Objective

1. To be able to participate in active games

Activities

1. There are so many active games that it isn't practical to try to give directions for teaching each one. Instead, general directions are given and should be adapted for the other games. Games include (but are not limited to): Ping-Pong, shuffleboard, darts, air hockey, badminton, horseshoes, lawn bowling, croquet.
2. First observe someone who knows the game playing it. Look at the implements used: racquets, paddles, balls, pucks, etc. Watch how the play begins, what each person does, how the turns are determined, how the players keep score, what ends the game. Write all this down on a chart when the group gets back to its room.
3. Get the appropriate implements for each person who wants to learn the game. Have participants practice the moves, hitting the ball, holding the paddle right, throwing the shoe, or whatever skills are needed. Give plenty of practice so that the person will have the skills before needing to learn how the game is played.
4. Practice starting the game and taking turns according to the style of the game. Do not bring up rules or scoring except to note that one isn't supposed to do it that way, or would do better another way.
5. Play a short game and introduce rules as they are needed. Don't introduce all the rules at once for it will be confusing. Don't keep score until everything above is fairly well mastered.
6. Introduce scoring last and deemphasize winning. People with very strong self-concepts may be able to handle competition, but others will be much more likely to stay involved with the game if it is played for fun.

Variations

1. Watch for possible presentations of the games on television.
2. If older adults play these games at a senior center, let one or two members of the group watch them play and, when they are ready, take part in the games.

Materials

1. Depending on the games, whatever paddles, racquets, balls, pucks, and so on are needed for the game

Lesson E: Collecting Antiques

Objectives

1. To be aware that people like old-fashioned things
2. To be able to respond to people who talk about or have valued antiques

Activities

1. Locate a few examples of old-fashioned things by asking someone who has a collection or a dealer. Things like clothing, tools, dolls, toys, and small items of furniture are appropriate. Show them to the group one at a time and talk about what they were used for. Locate them in time by saying that it was in "grandparents' " time or 100 years ago; keep it understandable.

2. Bring in or have the people in the group bring in the modern counterpart for each item, such as modern tools, toys, clothes. Talk about changes such as: less wood, more plastic; less hand decoration, more machine decoration. Ask if people have seen TV shows or movies about the old-fashioned days and if they can remember some ways the people in these shows lived differently from today's people: no refrigerators, no electric lights, no cars, no sewing machines, no washing machines, no TV, cooking on wood stove, making things by hand, amusing oneself without television, staying home more, canning food instead of freezing, and so forth.

3. Get books about antiques from the library or get magazines with pictures of them. Discuss this idea: When people get older, they remember how things used to be, they think of things they used to have, and they value old things. Many older adults are interested in collecting old things because these things remind them of when they were younger.

Variations

1. Go to a museum and look at the displays of antique furniture, dishes, clocks, machines, and other things that are too large to bring into a classroom.
2. Ask someone who has antiques in the home to invite a small group of interested participants to see them and hear about their history.

Materials

1. Old-fashioned items to display and the modern counterparts of each
2. Books and magazines about antiques

Lesson F: Taking Nature Walks or Hikes _____

Objectives

1. To be aware of nature hiking as a leisure activity
2. To know how to take a nature walk

Activities

1. Bring in some newspaper or magazine articles about hiking, local nature trails, scenery for which your area is known, anything about the outdoors that will introduce the subject of nature walks. Discuss these articles with the participants: who has seen the articles, who has done any nature hiking, who likes to be in the woods or on a trail?
2. Invite a member of a local hiking club or nature group to talk to the group about experiences. What makes hiking a good activity? Where does the person like to go? How does he/she prepare for a hike? What are the costs associated with it?
3. Get some old copies of *National Geographic* for browsing through. Have the participants look for pictures of scenery like they might see locally. Find pictures of people doing outdoor activities. Don't cut them out. Use other sports or nature magazines to cut from. Make a montage.
4. Gather brochures and schedules from local parks and scenic areas; visit them and take short walks. Come back and talk about what was seen. Gradually increase the length of the walks.
5. Talk about the kind of shoes and clothing one should wear for walking on trails instead of sidewalks or floors. Talk about what should be carried along and how much weight is enough to carry. Get everyone who wants to take a hike prepared for it and then take the hike.

Variations

1. Take a hike in town and see how much greenery and how many animals can be seen.
2. If there is a nature walking event or regular plan, participate in it. (One area park system has a program where those who take 10 hikes over the nature trails in the various parks can get a walking stick.)

Materials

1. News articles about hiking opportunities and schedules
2. Appropriate clothing and shoes for hiking
3. Brochures from local parks and scenic sites
4. *National Geographic* and other outdoor magazines

Lesson G: Enjoying Spectator Sports _____

Objectives

1. To know about the major spectator sports as leisure activities
2. To know about a sport the clients are going to watch, at least: the object of the game, what constitutes a score, and the name of the team they support

Activities

1. Spectator sports probably begin with watching television. If possible, videotape a game of:
    a. Baseball
    b. Basketball
    c. Soccer
    d. Tennis
    e. Football

    Study one game at a time. Suggest that nearly everyone needs to know a little about each game, and that each person can decide how much he/she wants to learn about each one. Make a chart of the following information. Watch a part of a game on videotape to find the answers or to illustrate the points if the answers are already known.

    • *What is the object of the game?*
    a. To make a hit and run the bases
    b. To throw the ball through the basket
    c. To kick the ball into the goal
    d. To hit the tennis ball so that the opponent cannot return it
    e. To get the ball across the goal line

    • *How does one side score against the other?*
    a. By hitting safely and running all the bases
    b. By making a basket or free throw
    c. By kicking or bumping the ball with any part of their bodies except the hands
    d. By hitting the ball so that it is inside the lines
    e. By carrying, throwing to a receiver, or kicking the ball over the goal line or through the goal posts

    • *What are the local teams called? (In one area, for example:)*
    a. Cleveland Indians
    b. Cleveland Cavaliers
    c. The Force
    d. No team
    e. Cleveland Browns

2. Using the information above, watch a game and have the people point out what is happening with regard to scoring and the object of the game. They should know whether the home team is winning or losing.

3. For those who want to know more about any or all of the sports, give information such as:
    a. Number of players on a team
    b. Number of points for each score
    c. Penalties, fouls, reasons some things that look like scores are not counted
    d. Time-outs—what they mean, what happens during one
    e. Names of leagues, other teams

4. Go to a local game at the high school and look for the things you know about the game. Find out the name of the home team and be aware of who wins the game.
5. Go to a professional game, and buy programs and save them for later use. When back in the room, look at the numbers of the players, pictures, statistics, and whatever else of interest is in the program.
6. If people are really interested in a sport, gather pictures of favorite players and make a Hall of Fame for the room.

Variations

1. Listen to a game on radio; when the announcer uses various specialized terms, explain what they mean.
2. Make a display of sports balls: football, baseball, basketball, soccer ball, tennis ball. Play a game in which one person names either a team or a player and the other must pick up the right ball for that sport.

Materials

1. Videotapes of major sports games, preferably featuring local professional teams
2. Chart paper, felt markers
3. Photos of players, teams
4. Various kinds of sports balls: football, basketball, baseball, soccer ball, tennis ball

Lesson H: Singing

Objectives

1. To be aware of singing as a leisure activity
2. To be able to sing some commonly known songs

Activities

1. Play several records of folk songs or the old songs everyone knows. Stop after each one and talk about it; try to hum along with the tune. Decide which one(s) people want to learn.
2. Have the words to the songs printed for those who want to use them. Give them to everyone and go over them several times. Invite a guitar player to accompany the group as they learn to put words and music together.
3. Songs that most older people know can be identified by contacting a senior center or local glee club. Ask someone to come and sing the songs with the group to get them ready to participate in sing-alongs. Explain that senior citizen groups often have sing-alongs for entertainment.
4. Tape record the singing and have a cassette available for anyone who wants to perfect the tune or words to use individually.
5. Invite other workshop staff to participate in a song show just before work starts or during lunch time.

Variations

1. Go to a performance of a high school glee club or other local singing group.
2. Attend a gospel sing or performance at a local church.

Materials

1. Records of the "old songs"
2. Words to the songs

Lesson I: Visiting a Museum

Objectives

1. To know that museums are places where one goes in leisure time
2. To be able to find a specific exhibit in a museum

Activities

1. Start this unit when there is a special exhibit coming to the museum and publicity is appearing in newspaper. Cut out the articles and display them. Discuss the special exhibit, and, if there is interest, take the participants to see it.
2. If there is no special exhibit, build motivation by linking this to another teaching activity (for example, after studying antiques, go to the museum to see an antiques exhibit).
3. Get a floor plan and descriptions of displays from a museum. In the classroom, make either a transparency or an enlarged map on chart paper. With the group, label each section and discuss what might be found there. If possible, use postcards from the museum that portray specific items on exhibit in that area. Put them on the room where they will be found.
4. Using the postcards or pictures (taken by the leader) of displays, decide with the group what is of most interest to them. Get whatever information is available about what will be seen. Some museums sell slides or have tape cassettes that could be borrowed for this use. Tell the group what they will see before going. Go to the museum and, while there, point out the displays mentioned. After the trip, remember with the group what was seen. Talk about it BEFORE—DURING—AFTER.
5. Go to only one section at a time so that the participants will be able to enjoy and appreciate what they were prepared to see instead of just having a hazy memory of walking past a lot of unrelated exhibits.

Variations

1. Many libraries have exhibits of local history that might be interesting.
2. Ask the museum director if there are speakers who might come and talk to the group about either the whole museum or special displays.
3. Specialty museums may be in the area. For example, there are museums of health, transportation, natural history, state history, and history of specific local industry.

Materials

1. Brochures, floor plans, descriptions from museums
2. Publicity about special exhibits

Lesson J: Going Camping

Objectives

1. To be able to enjoy being away from home overnight
2. To get as close to real camping as can be tolerated and enjoyed

Activities

1. Most older adults are not enthusiastic about real camping, in which they would sleep in sleeping bags on the ground and cook over open fires. Modify the experience to meet their needs and desires. It is possible to go away from home overnight, do outdoor activities, and eat foods cooked outdoors without "roughing it."
2. Before you present camping to the group, have some idea of how the plan will work. If you can use a camper or van for sleeping, know where it will be procured. You might want to stay in cabins or lodge at a state park. Also get the prices for some motels near the area where you might go. Participants probably can afford shared rooms. Locate some camping cookers that use propane gas or charcoal.
3. Present the idea of taking an overnight trip to see a natural or scenic place. Have brochures available to look at. If anyone has been to one of these places, ask him/her to bring pictures or souvenirs to show. The group should decide where to go, and choose from the alternative places to sleep and eat.
4. Plan very thoroughly what to take, what to wear, and what activities will be done at the chosen site. Assign responsibilities to individuals. Take the trip. Afterward, evaluate the experience and decide what needs to be considered when taking other trips in the future.

Variations

1. City "camping"—camp out in a city motel and explore the sights of the town after doing the same kind of advance planning as above.
2. Start with a day camp experience in which outdoor cooking is tested.

Materials

1. Brochures, pictures, souvenirs of nature or scenic sights
2. Information about possible lodges, motels, or sleeping accommodations
3. Outdoor cooking stove and fuel

Lesson K: Participating in Travelogues

Objectives

1. To be able to participate in viewing travelogues
2. To know how to react to travelogues as others expect

Activities

1. Motivate study of the new topic by telling the group that you will be learning how people learn about faraway places and other kinds of people in the world. Talk about travel programs they may have seen on television. Ask who has taken a trip anywhere and find out if they took photos to remember it by.
2. Collect and bring in travel magazines such as *National Geographic* and make them available to look through. Try to find pictures of places and people who look familiar or who are quite different. If the magazines can be cut up, make a montage of pictures cut out by the members of the group.
3. Ask the members to bring in photos from trips they have taken. Ask staff to do the same; make a display or show the photos one at a time.
4. Invite someone from the community to show slides of a trip. Just show the pictures and don't talk too much about each one other than to say what it shows. Respond to questions, but don't elaborate.
5. Select a specific place to focus on. Have travel pictures shown; bring in art objects, costumes, souvenirs, or other materials from that place. If someone is from there, have them tell the group about it and answer questions.
6. Discuss the appropriate kinds of comments one makes about travelogues and practice making them.
7. Go to a public presentation of a travelogue in the community, preparing for it in advance and discussing it afterwards.

Variations

1. Play mood music for a travelogue by getting tapes or records of the appropriate area's music.
2. If people are interested, show them where the places are on a map.
3. Listen to tapes or records of different languages.

Materials

1. Magazines with travel pictures
2. Slides, films, photos of other places
3. Posters, art objects, souvenirs, costumes from other places

Unit XVII. Exercises

Lesson A: Motivation to Exercise

Objectives

1. To strengthen heart, lungs, muscles, and all body systems
2. To stay active and healthy
3. To know exercises that might be done in community settings

Activities

1. As a group, watch an exercise show on television, or get a videotape of exercises (not aerobic). Look for one that is for older adults. After watching the program, discuss the reasons for exercising regularly, including: losing weight, making muscles stronger, helping circulation, deep breathing, just feeling good.
2. Invite someone who practices regular exercising to talk to the group about what benefits can be obtained from this activity. Talk about how that person decided to do it, what it costs, how often it is done, where, and with whom. Give time for questions.
3. Ask the group to be ready to tell how much exercise they get now and how often they do it. Figure out how much of the day is spent sitting, lying down, and moving. Ask some very active staff from the workshop to calculate the same things and compare them.
4. Suggest that everyone should participate in daily exercise with the group. Some may want to go into it more, and they will learn other exercises and have scheduled time to do them with others. Note that exercise programs are often part of the daily schedule at senior centers, and that knowing how to do exercises in advance will make it easier to participate when clients go to a center.
5. Collect and display articles and pictures about exercising from magazines. Look for short films and records to use with nonaerobic exercises. Take photos of individual group members doing exercises.
6. Lead the group or get a volunteer to lead daily exercises for everyone. After the warm-up exercise period, provide time for the ones who want to do more. Do the exercises to music to help the participants follow the rhythms.

Variations

1. Enroll several members in exercise programs at the Y or civic center, especially if they are suitable for older adults.
2. Ask several high school athletes of both sexes to demonstrate and lead exercises for your group.
3. Exercise in a swimming pool so that there will be less stress on foot and leg muscles.

Materials

1. Books, magazine articles, photos, pictures of people exercising
2. Exercise videotapes, records, cassettes
3. Records or cassettes to use during exercise periods

Lesson B: Suggested Senior Exercises* _____

These exercises are only suggested. If there are reasons participants cannot do certain ones, then they should be modified or eliminated. Instruct class members that if at any time they experience any trembling, nausea, extreme breathlessness, pounding in the head, or pain in the chest, they should **stop** immediately. These are signs that they have reached their level of exercise tolerance. Gauge the number of repetitions to do by the general ability of the class. It is easier and safer when doing standing exercises to hold onto a chair for balance. The following abbreviations are used throughout the exercise directions: SP = starting position; R = right; L = left.

Sitting

1. Sit up nice and straight and relax. Inhale, place your arms over head, and stretch. Repeat.
2. Reach for the sky and sway side to side, stretching.
3. Reaching for the sky—arms go side to side like an airplane.
4. Touch floor (or near it) bending side to side.
5. Side bend—one hand over head, hold stretch.
6. Leg lifts—lift one leg 6 times, switch, repeat; total 12 leg lifts each leg.
7. Circle ankle—reverse directions (one at a time).
8. Arm circles palms up—small circles forward and back.
9. Leg raise—raise legs up and down; point toes toward front, heels together.
10. Arm circles palms down—small circles, forward and back.
11. Arms outstretched, touch shoulders, touch sky, touch shoulders—arms outstretched, twist palms up and down—repeat 3 times saying "in, up, out, twist, twist."
12. (Similar to above) Arms stretched out in front, touch shoulders, touch sky stretch, touch shoulders, finish arms outstretched in front—twist palms 2 times. Repeat three times saying "in, up, in, forward, twist, twist."
13. Cross arms over chest (shoulder high), double twist to each side.
14. Back crawl—pretend to swim.
15. Front crawl
16. Hands on shoulders, circle elbows, reverse.
17. Hands on shoulders, touch elbows together.
18. Hands on shoulders, touch opposite knee to elbow.
19. Push up one arm overhead 6–8 repetitions, switch and do other arm.
20. Push up both arms overhead.
21. Push arms straight out in front from shoulders, then pull back, bringing hands to shoulders (like rowing a boat).
22. Rotate shoulders forward, then back.
23. Arms overhead, hands together, reach back as far as possible (stretching rib cage).
24. Head, look side to side (like saying "no").
25. Head, touch ear to shoulder (like saying "maybe").
26. Head, chin to chest, look up at ceiling (like saying "yes").
27. Head rolls nice and easy all the way around, reverse.
28. *Crossovers with Arms*—cross one arm over the other back and forth fast and reverse.
29. "Pick apples," reaching up with one arm, then the other.

_____

*Taken from Herrera, P. (1983). *Innovative programming for the aging & aged mentally retarded/developmentally disabled adult*. Akron, OH: Exploration Press.

30. Reach arms up over head, touch knees, then toes, then knees and repeat.
31. Circle wrists and reverse.
32. Pretend you're playing the piano.
33. Pretend you're boxing.
34. Tap each finger to thumb and back again (one tap, then two taps, etc.).
35. Holding hands over head, sway side to side.
36. *Single-Leg Bicycle*—using arms for support, bring one knee up to chest, return to outstretched position and bring other leg up. Alternate quickly.
37. *Double-Leg Bicycle*—sitting with legs straight, bend knees and bring feet toward rear end and return. Work up to not touching floor in between.
38. *Knees In, Up, Down*—bring knees in as in #37, but lift both feet up in air as high as possible, then lower slowly to floor.
39. *Crossovers*—using arms for support (as you get stronger, do not use arms), lift legs up in the air. Spread legs apart, then cross L leg over R leg, spread, then cross R leg over L leg.
40. *Flutter Kick*—with legs straight and toes pointed, lift legs off ground and kick up and down using the entire leg. Don't touch floor. Do for a count or a length of time.
41. *Leg to Side*—with legs stretched out in front, swing one leg to the side as far as possible, return to SP and repeat.
42. *Alternating Leg Crossovers*—in same SP as #41, lift one leg up and cross over body to other side. Return to SP and cross other leg over.
43. *Straddle Reach*—with legs spread apart and straight, reach R hand to left foot, then L hand to R foot.
44. *Head-to-Knee Stretch*—same SP as #43; stretch head to one knee, hold 5 seconds, stretch to other side and hold.
45. *Head-to-Middle Stretch*—same SP as #44; stretch head down to floor between legs. Hold. Repeat. *Do Not Bounce!*
46. *Lower Back Stretch*—place soles of feet together, grasp toes, and pull head toward feet. Hold 5 seconds and relax.
47. *Inner Thigh Stretch*—same SP as #46; grasp ankles with hands and place elbows on the inside of the knees. Push down knees with elbows and hold for 5 seconds. Relax.
48. *Arch and Reach*—with legs straight out in front and arms slightly behind hips, lift hips off floor, lower; then reach toward feet while keeping legs straight.
49. *Walking Feet*—sit with knees bent, grab toes with arms outside legs, and walk feet as far out in front as possible. Hold for 5 seconds and walk back.
50. *Pikes*—with legs stretched out in front, simultaneously lift legs up and bring arms out in front to touch ankles. Return almost to SP, but do not let legs touch floor.
51. *Single Knee Bend, Lift, Lower*—with legs stretched out in front, bring one knee in toward body, lift leg in air, and slowly lower to ground. Do other leg. Alternate back and forth.
52. *Four-Count Leg Lower*—with legs out in front, bring both knees up to chest. Lift up in air, lower till 6 inches off ground, and hold for 4 counts; spread legs apart and hold for 4 counts; bring legs back together and hold for 4 counts. Return to SP and repeat sequence.

Standing

1. *Butterflies*—rotate both arms forward, reverse (or one arm at a time).
2. *Head Rolls*—roll head slowly one direction. Switch directions.
3. *Shoulder Shrugs*—lift and rotate shoulders up and forward. Reverse.

4. *Trunk Twist*—hands on hips, rotate trunk to L, then R. Stretch.

5. *Side Bends*—one hand on hip with other hand stretched overhead, stretch to the L, then repeat to the R. Hold stretch each side for 20 seconds.

6. *Reach for the Sky*—bring both hands up over head, come up on toes, and stretch as high as possible. Or do one hand at a time.

7. *Knee Pulls*—pull one knee up to chest, keeping toe pointed and back straight. Switch legs.

8. *Toe Raises*—rise up and down on toes. Point them toward the front, out to the side, and turn them in.

9. *Arm Circles*—extend arms out to side at shoulder level, and make small circles, gradually increasing to large circles. Reverse.

10. *Swimming*—Pretend to do the crawl stroke with arms. Reverse.

11. *Touch Shoulders*
    a. Reach up and down from shoulders—extend arms.
    b. Reach out to side from shoulders and back.
    c. Reach out in front and return—keep elbows shoulder level.

12. *Windmills*—with feet a shoulder-width apart, touch R hand to L foot, then L hand to R foot. Return to standing position each time.

13. *Head to Knee*—with feet a shoulder-width apart, grasp ankle or lower leg and pull head as close to knee as possible. Hold 5 seconds. Repeat to other side.

14. *Waist Twist*—with hands extended to side at shoulder level, twist waist R then to L.

15. *Pull Foot to Hip*—facing a wall for support, reach back and grasp foot, pull towards hip. Switch legs.

16. *Leg Stretch*—grasp inside of foot and straighten leg to side.

17. *Wall Push-Aways*—standing about 3 feet from wall, hands about shoulder level, bend elbows and lean into wall. Push back to SP.

18. *Mountain Climbing*—squat down and place hands in front of body on floor with one leg stretched out behind and the other leg bent under the chest. Rapidly switch position of the legs.

19. *Knee Bends*—with hands on hips, bend knees and squat toward ground. Go only about halfway down.

20. *Jumping Jacks*—begin standing with arms at side. Simultaneously raise hands over head and spread legs apart. Return to SP.

21. *Kicks*
    a. In front—kick leg in front as far as possible.
    b. Behind—kick leg behind as far as possible.
    c. Side—lift leg to side up and down.

22. *Standing Leg Circles*—stretch leg out to side and circle leg. Increase size of circle and reverse direction.

23. *Jog in Place*—jog for a count or a period of time in one place.

24. *Wall Sit*—with back facing wall, slide down the wall until legs are bent at a right angle. Hold that position. Increase length of hold.

25. *Golf Swing*—with feet a shoulder-width apart, swing both arms together up to side as far as possible. Swing to other side.

26. *Reverse Squats*—with feet about 12–15 inches apart, squat down so hands are on floor. Leaving hands in place, straighten legs. Return to SP.

27. *In front, middle, behind touches*—with feet a shoulder-width apart, reach down and touch the floor in front of feet, between feet, and behind feet as far as possible.

28. *Sweeping Circles*—with hands together and arms straight, make a large circle sweeping floor with hands and reaching above head.

PART 2

Instructor's Guide

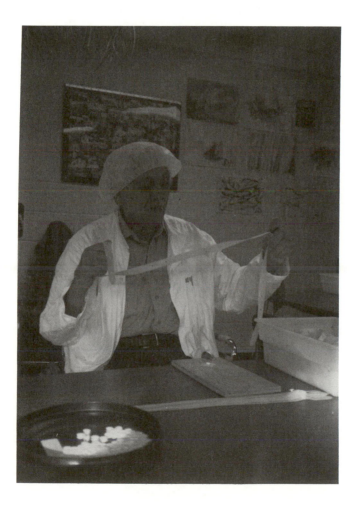

Introduction

The *Instructor's Guide* is intended to be used with the primary text, *Expanding Options for Older Adults with Developmental Disabilities*. It is a guide for the instructor in presenting the text material and assisting trainees in learning the concepts presented in the text.

The *Guide* is divided into sections, each corresponding to a section in the text. These are:

Section I: Normal Aging
Section II: Nature and Needs of Elderly Persons with Mental Retardation/Developmental Disabilities
Section III: Planning for Community Access
Section IV: Discipline with Dignity: How to Work with Dependent Adults
Section V: Meeting the Unique Needs of Individuals: The Interdisciplinary Process

Each section in the *Instructor's Guide* includes a list of competencies and objectives to be attained by trainees. Detailed lesson plans for each session are presented. Each plan includes activities of the trainer/instructor and the trainees or students. They closely follow the text materials that are basic to each session.

Lecture outlines accompany the lesson plan for each session. Detailed instructions for conducting special learning activities are given. Handouts that may be copied for the training group are included.

The lesson plans for each of the five sections are comprehensive and geared to a total of 6 to 8 hours of training for each section. However, the instructor can select those lectures, films, and activities that best meet needs of the trainees and fit time limitations of the training event. The *Instructor's Guide* is intended to be a flexible tool. Instructors are encouraged to be creative and to make modifications and adaptations.

THE INSTRUCTOR

Instructors using this guide must be very familiar with the text, *Expanding Options for Older Adults with Developmental Disabilities*. Some time will need to be invested in studying the section that will be presented, as well as appropriate references. Guest speakers who are experts in a specific topic within the lesson plan may be utilized if the instructor does not feel comfortable with the subject.

It is essential that the instructor be knowledgeable about developmentally disabled older people and other dependent adults who are the primary focus of the text and the *Instructor's Guide*.

A basic understanding of principles of adult education is desirable. Some background in teaching and/or public speaking, group leadership, or other related experiences is needed. The instructor should understand the importance of a variety of teaching methods such as lectures, discussion, group process, simulation, role play, visual aids, and so forth.

Above all, the instructor must have commitment to the principles and concepts included in the text, especially those presented in Sections IV and V.

TRAINEES

Those to be trained may include any professional staff person, volunteer, or family member who has ongoing contact with developmentally disabled older adults or other dependent adults in restricted settings, such as nursing homes or retirement centers. Professionals and service providers from the network of services to the aging will also find many of the sessions useful.

Normal Aging

COMPETENCIES

I. Knowledge: Trainees will know and be able to discuss
   A. Demographic trends in the "graying of America"
   B. Historical factors affecting the status of older persons in American society
   C. Dimensions of aging, including
      1. Biological
      2. Psychological
      3. Social
   D. Interventions that can prevent or mitigate negative effects of normal aging
   E. Options in living arrangements for older adults
   F. Income and work changes with aging
   G. Leisure and recreational preferences of older persons
   H. Community services provided by the Older Americans Act and by various organizations/agencies
   I. Definitions of relevant terminology
II. Skills: Trainees will be able to
   A. Recognize and refute myths about aging persons
   B. Locate information about aging
   C. Identify community services that can be accessed by older adults
III. Attitude: Trainees will
   A. Focus on the strengths and assets of older adults when planning activities for them
   B. Seek out normalizing, integrated settings for older adults with developmental disabilities

OBJECTIVES

I. Trainees will be able to
   A. Define gerontology and geriatrics
   B. List six stereotypes of aging
   C. Describe demographic trends in aging over the years 1900–2010
   D. Define terms: "young-old" and "old-old"
   E. Identify five states with high density of older adult population; two with lowest
   F. Define "well elderly," "frail elderly," and "institutionalized elderly"
   G. Describe a minimum of six changes in the physiology of older adults
   H. Identify changes over the life span in
      1. Memory
      2. Intelligence

3. Learning
4. Personality
    as these are now viewed by gerontologists

I. Discuss role loss and role assignment as these apply to the older population
J. List five possible roles in later life
K. List six options for living arrangements during the later years
L. Illustrate by graph drawing changes in income that occur with retirement
M. Define the Older Americans Act
N. List eight community services specifically provided for older adults
O. Describe the concept of formal and informal support systems

LESSON PLAN, SESSION 1: INTRODUCTION TO NORMAL AGING

Competencies: I (A): Trainees will know and be able to discuss demographic trends in the "graying" of America
I (B): Trainees will know and be able to discuss historical factors affecting the status of older persons in American society

Objectives: I (A): Trainees will be able to define gerontology and geriatrics
I (B): Trainees will be able to list six stereotypes of aging
I (C): Trainees will be able to describe demographic trends in aging over the years 1900–2010
I (D): Trainees will be able to define terms: "young-old" and "old-old"
I (E): Trainees will be able to identify five states with high density of older adult population; two with lowest
I (F): Trainees will be able to define "well elderly," "frail elderly," and "institutionalized elderly"

Instructor	Trainee	Materials
Present information on terminology, definitions (Lecture Outline 1.I)	Take notes or underline text Discuss—What would you prefer to be called as an older person?	Primary text, Chapter 1
Hand out and explain the quiz	Write answers to quiz	Quiz: "Facts on Aging"
Lead discussion on answers to quiz; emphasize myths; distribute Handout 1: "Life-Style Changes"	Participate in discussion—answer	Handout 1: "Life-Style Changes"
Present demographic information about older population (Lecture Outline 1.II)		Primary text, Chapter 1; transparencies or blow-ups of Figure 1.1 and Table 1.1
Present information on the history of aging in America (Lecture Outline 1.III)	Take notes or underline text	Primary text, Chapter 1

Evaluation: Answers to quiz questions

LECTURE OUTLINE 1: INTRODUCTION

I.   Terminology
    A.   Gerontology: the multidisciplinary study of aging
        1.   Draws from many disciplines
            a.   Sociology
            b.   Psychology
            c.   Biology
            d.   Economics
            e.   History, political science
            f.   The arts
            g.   Others
    B.   Geriatrics: the specialized field of medicine that is concerned with the elderly
        1.   Comparatively new to the United States
            a.   Few trained geriatricians
            b.   Few medical schools with specialized studies
        2.   Europe, Great Britain, Canada, more experienced
    C.   The older population can be subdivided into
        1.   Young-old (65–74)
        2.   Middle-old (75–84)
        3.   Old-old (85 +)
II. Demographics of aging
    A.   Growth in past decades
    B.   Projected growth
    C.   Sex ratio
    D.   Over 85, fastest growing segment of population
    E.   Ratio of elderly to teenagers
    F.   Effects of infant mortality, technology, the Depression, baby boom, on present and future statistics
    G.   States with greatest numbers of older residents
III. History of aging in America
    A.   Colonial America
        1.   Importance of agriculture, trade, religion, family
        2.   Age hierarchy
        3.   Uncle Sam
        4.   Older people were needed: concept of developing country
    B.   Industrial Revolution
        1.   Technology; obsolete skills
        2.   Rush to the cities; overcrowding; poverty
        3.   Development of "speed up"
        4.   Changes in social thought, values
    C.   The elderly as a social problem, Civil War–1900s
        1.   Poorhouses
        2.   Rolelessness
        3.   No pension system
        4.   Old age as a disease
    D.   Significance of Social Security Act, 1935
        1.   Retirement
        2.   Social Security payments: a supplement
        3.   Labels, myths of aging
        4.   Segregated housing; visibility of the aged

FACTS ON AGING

T F 1. The majority of old people (past age 65) are senile (i.e., defective memory, disoriented, or demented).

T F 2. All five senses tend to decline in old age.

T F 3. Most old people have no interest in, or capacity for, sexual relations.

T F 4. Lung capacity tends to decline in old age.

T F 5. The majority of old people feel miserable most of the time.

T F 6. Physical strength tends to decline in old age.

T F 7. At least one tenth of the aged are living in long-stay institutions (e.g., nursing homes, mental hospitals, homes for the aged)

T F 8. Aged drivers have fewer accidents per person than drivers under age 65.

T F 9. Most older workers cannot work as effectively as younger workers.

T F 10. About 80% of the aged are healthy enough to carry out their normal activities.

T F 11. Most old people are set in their ways and unable to change.

T F 12. Old people usually take longer to learn something new.

T F 13. It is almost impossible for most old people to learn new things.

T F 14. The reaction time of most old people tends to be slower than reaction time of younger people.

T F 15. In general, most old people are pretty much alike.

T F 16. The majority of old people are seldom bored.

T F 17. The majority of old people are socially isolated and lonely.

T F 18. Older workers have fewer accidents than younger workers.

T F 19. Over 15% of the U.S. population are now age 65 or over.

T F 20. Most medical practitioners tend to give low priority to the aged.

T F 21. The majority of older people have incomes below the poverty level (as defined by the federal government).

T F 22. The majority of old people are working or would like to have some kind of work to do (including housework and volunteer work).

T F 23. Older people tend to become more religious as they age.

T F 24. The majority of old people are seldom irritated or angry.

T F 25. The health and socioeconomic status of older people (compared to younger people) in the year 2000 will probably be about the same as now.

Developed by Erdman Palmore (1977) at the Center for the Study of Aging and Human Development at the Duke University Medical Center.

91

ANSWERS TO FACTS ON AGING QUIZ

Note: The key to the correct answers is simple: all the odd-numbered items are false and all the even-numbered are true.

1. False. The majority of old people are not senile. Cognitive function shows both increase and decrease across the life span depending on the processes involved. Only about 2% of people over 65 are institutionalized as a result of psychiatric illness. All the evidence indicates that there are less than 10% of the aged who are disoriented or demented.

2. True. All five senses tend to decline in old age. Most studies agree that various aspects of vision, hearing, touch, taste, and smell tend to decline in old age.

3. False. The majority of people past age 65 continue to have both interest in, and capacity for, sexual relations. Masters and Johnson[1] found that the capacity for satisfying sexual relations continues into the decades of the 70s and 80s for healthy couples.

4. True. Lung capacity does tend to decline in old age. In fact, maximum breathing capacity declines on the average from age 30 onward.

5. False. The majority of old people do not feel miserable most of the time. Studies of happiness, morale, and life satisfaction find no significant difference by age groups— or find about one fifth to one third of the aged score "low" on various happiness or morale scales.

6. True. Physical strength does tend to decline in age.

7. False. Only 4.8% of people 65 and over were residents of any long-stay institutions in 1970 (U.S. Census). Even among those age 75 or over, only 9.2% were residents of institutions.

8. True. Drivers over age 65 have fewer accidents per person than drivers under age 65; however, they also drive fewer miles per year. Older drivers have about the same accident rate per person as middle-aged drivers, but a much lower rate than drivers under age 30.

9. False. The majority of older workers can work as efficiently as younger workers. Despite declines in perception and reaction speed under laboratory conditions among the general aged population, studies of older workers under actual working conditions show that they perform as well as, if not better than, younger workers, most of the time. Consistency of output tends to increase with age, as older workers perform at steadier rates from week to week than younger workers do. In addition, older workers have less job turnover, fewer accidents, and less absenteeism than younger workers.

10. True. About 80% of the aged are healthy enough to engage in normal activities. About 5% of those over age 65 are institutionalized and another 15% among the non-institutionalized say they are unable to engage in their major activities because of chronic conditions.

11. False. The majority of old people are not set in their ways and unable to change. Older people tend to become more stable in their attitudes, but it is clear that most older people do change and adapt to the many major life events that occur in old age. Their political and social attitudes also tend to shift with those of the rest of society, although at a somewhat slower rate than for younger people. The idea that older people are more "rigid" is not supported by the research literature.

12. True. Old people usually take longer to learn something new, but it is not impossible for most old people to learn new things.

13. False. Older people can usually learn anything anyone else can if given enough time and/or well-designed learning approaches.

14. True. Young people do have a faster reaction time than old people. This is one of the best documented facts about the aged on record. It appears to be true regardless of the kind of reaction that is measured.

15. False. Most old people are not alike; in fact, evidence indicates that as people age they tend to become less alike and more heterogeneous on many dimensions.

16. True. The majority of old people are seldom bored. Only 17% of people 65 or over say "not enough to do to keep busy" is a "somewhat serious" or "very serious" problem.

17. False. The majority of old people are not socially isolated and lonely. About two thirds of the aged say they are never or hardly ever lonely. Most older persons have close relatives within easy visiting distance, and contact between them is relatively frequent. Between visits with relatives and friends and participation in church and other voluntary organizations, the majority of old people are far from socially isolated.

18. True. Older workers have fewer accidents than younger workers. Most studies support this as true. In one major study workers beyond age 65 had about one half the rate of nondisabling injuries as those under 65, and older workers have lower rates of disabling injuries.

19. False. In 1975, 10.3% of the population was age 65 or over. At the beginning of 1980 the estimated 25 million older Americans made up over 11% of the population— "every ninth American." This will probably increase to over 12% by the year 2000, even if population growth drops to zero.

20. True. Most medical practitioners tend to give low priority to the aged. A series of 12 empirical studies found that most medical students and doctors, nursing students and nurses, occupational therapy students, psychiatry clinic personnel, and social workers tend to believe the negative stereotypes about the aged and prefer to work with children or younger adults rather than with the aged. Few specialize, or are interested in specializing, in geriatrics.

21. False. In 1975, 15.3% of people over 65 were below the official poverty level (about $2,400 for an individual or $3,000 for a couple). If the "near-poor" are included, the total in or near poverty is 25.4%. However, most people 65 or over have incomes well above the poverty level. Women and minority members are heavily overrepresented among the aged poor.

22. True. Over three fourths of old people are working or would like to have some kind of work to do. About 12% of those 65 or over are employed; 21% are retired but say they would like to be employed; 17% work as housekeepers; 19% are not employed but do volunteer work; and another 9% are not employed and not doing volunteer work but would like to do volunteer work. These percentages total 78%.

23. False. Older people do not tend to become more religious as they age. While it is true that the present generation of older people tends to be more religious than the younger generations, this appears to be a generational difference rather than an aging effect, resulting from the upbringing of the older person.

24. True. The majority of old people are seldom irritated or angry. The Kansas City Study found that over one half the aged said they are never or hardly ever irritated and this proportion increases to two thirds at age 80 or over.

25. False. The health and socioeconomic status of older people, compared with younger people, in the year 2000 will probably be much higher than now. Measures of health, income, occupation, and education among older people are all rising in comparison with those of younger people.

REFERENCE

[1] Masters, W. M., & Johnson, V. E. (1966). *Human sexual response*. Boston: Little, Brown.

LIFE-STYLE CHANGES: MEETING THE CHALLENGE

It is not by muscle, speed, or physical dexterity that great things are achieved, but by reflection, force of character and judgement. In these qualities old age is not poorer, but is even richer.

—Cicero (106–43 B.C.)

To be seventy years young is sometimes far more cheerful and hopeful than to be forty years old.

—Oliver Wendell Holmes

COMMON MYTHS ON AGING

1. To be OLD is to be SENILE
2. To be OLD is to be DYING
3. To be OLD is to be LONELY
4. To be OLD is to be DEPRESSED
5. To be OLD is to be SEXUALLY IMPOTENT
6. To be OLD is to be BORED
7. To be OLD is to be USELESS
8. To be OLD is to be a HYPOCHONDRIAC
9. To be OLD is to go DOWNHILL
10. To be OLD is to be UNPRODUCTIVE

Nothing is more beautiful than cheerfulness in an old face.

—Richter

THE CHALLENGE OF GROWING OLDER

1. Changing roles
2. Changing family patterns, friendships, and other social networks
3. Changing economic status
4. Changing behaviors in mind and body
5. Changing interests and opportunities

From Moshe Torem, M.D.

LESSON PLAN, SESSION 2: BIOLOGICAL CHANGES

Competency: I (C-1): Trainees will know and be able to discuss biological dimensions of aging
I (D): Trainees will know and be able to discuss interventions that can prevent or mitigate negative effects of normal aging
Objectives: I (G): Trainees will be able to describe a minimum of six changes in the physiology of older adults

Instructor	Trainee	Materials
Organize small groups to discuss obvious physiological/biological changes that occur with age	Participate in small group discussion	
Lead general discussion of small group reports; emphasize *interventions* that can offset these changes; emphasize sensory losses	Report observations to class as a whole Listen to record (or participate in other sensory-loss sensitivity exercise) Discuss "which sensory loss would be worse to experience"	Recording of distorted sound, or other sensory-loss sensitivity activity (e.g., blindfolding)
Discuss effects of environmental, social, and political factors on health and physical condition of older adults in the past and in contemporary society; distribute Activity Handout 1: "Then and Now"	Participate in discussion; do activity	Leader's instructions, Activity 1: "Influences on Health and Physical Condition"; copies of Activity Handout 1: "Then and Now"
Present information on changes in nervous system, cardiovascular system, bone structure and other possible changes; present health continuum and biological theories of aging (Lecture Outline 2)	Take notes Ask questions Participate in discussion	Primary text, Chapter 2; transparency or blow-up of Figure 2.1
Select an activity from Activity 2: "Biological Changes"	Participate in activity	Leader's instructions, Activity 2: "Biological Changes"; sets of photos of stages of life, mounted sequentially; pictures from magazines, mounting paper, paste or glue (see activity sheet)

Evaluation: List major new information learned

LECTURE OUTLINE 2: BIOLOGICAL CHANGES

    I.   All biological systems undergo change over the life span
        A.   Cardiovascular
        B.   Bone
        C.   Nervous
        D.   Endocrine
        E.   Sensory
        F.   Immune system
   II.   Visible changes over the life span
  III.   Other changes
  IV.   Many changes can be prevented, modified, or reversed by
        A.   Transplants and replacements
        B.   Exercise
        C.   Medication
            1.   For example, osteoporosis can be prevented by calcium and estrogen
        D.   Diet, nutrition
        E.   Other: cosmetic, prosthetic
   V.   Most diseases and conditions of the elderly are chronic
        A.   Examples: arthritis, diabetes, heart disease, vision and hearing deficiencies
        B.   Treatment
  VI.   Health viewed on a continuum
 VII.   Self-report of the elderly
        A.   Noninterference of health conditions with activity
        B.   Percentages: well elderly, 80%; frail, 10%–15%; institutionalized, 4%–5%

INFLUENCES ON HEALTH AND PHYSICAL CONDITION
(Leader's Instructions)

Purpose

1. To compare the environments in which different generations were raised
2. To consider the effects of the different conditions upon the physical condition of people who were young in other eras

Activities

1. Divide the class into small groups of four or five people and give each group a copy of Activity Handout 1.
2. Ask participants to remember conditions as they were in the 1920s or 1930s, before World War II. They may need to remember movies or documentaries they have seen.
3. Have participants complete the handout and be ready to contribute to the group discussion. What were the conditions and how did they contribute to the physical health of children growing up in that era?
4. In each group, discuss whether children today are in a better or less healthful environment.

Materials

1. Enough copies of Activity Handout 1 for each person or group

THEN AND NOW

Think about the different kinds of lives people who are now old have experienced as compared to the kind that younger people are experiencing. These people were young in the 1920s, adolescent in the 1930s, and middle-aged in the 1950s and 1960s.

Using the format below, list influences in each category that might affect health status for each age group.

Influences on Health and Physical Condition

	Old Now	Young Now
Economic Conditions		
Nutrition		
Residence		
Exercise		
Medical Care		
Dental Care		
Epidemics		
Contagious Diseases		
Daily Schedules		
Agencies Available		

Come back together as a whole group and discuss your lists.

BIOLOGICAL CHANGES (Leader's Instructions)

Purpose

1. To observe that all living things go through a natural sequence from youth to old age
2. To discuss the assets and liabilities of each phase of life
3. To relate phases of life to specific persons known

Activities

1. Have on display photo sets of living things at various stages of life:
    a. Roses from bud to full bloom to "last rose of summer"
    b. Cats from kitten to mature to old cat
    c. People from infant to child to adult to old person
2. Have pictures cut from magazines available, and have small groups make montages illustrating the flow of life.
3. For each stage of life, discuss and list on chart or chalkboard:
    a. Assets of each stage of life
    b. Liabilities, weaknesses, stresses of each stage
4. Have each person think of someone who is old now and try to remember or picture that person as a baby, child, youth, adult.

Materials

1. Sets of pictures of plants, animals, people at different stages of life mounted sequentially
2. Pictures from magazines showing people at different stages of life; mounting paper to make a montage; paste or glue

LESSON PLAN, SESSION 3: PSYCHOLOGICAL CHANGES

Competency: I (C-2): Trainees will know and be able to discuss psychological dimensions of aging
Objective: I (H): Trainees will be able to identify changes over the life span in memory, intelligence, learning, and personality

Instructor	Trainee	Materials
Lead discussion on common myths of mental functioning in the later years	Participate in discussion	Primary text, Chapter 2
Develop list of myths (on chalkboard)	Develop list	Chalkboard or flipchart
Present information about current research on intelligence, learning, and memory and aging process (Lecture Outline 3A)	Take notes or underline text	Primary text, Chapter 2
Show movie: *Aging*	View film; discuss	Film: *Aging* (see Audiovisual Resources, p. 114); projector and screen
Lead discussion about film: Refer to list of personality types in Chapter 2 (p. 13)		Transparency or blow-up of Table 2.1
Present information on pathological conditions (Lecture Outline 3B)	Take notes or underline text Ask questions	Primary text, Chapter 2
Distribute Activity Handout 1: "Personality Patterns"	Participate; follow instructions on activity handout	Activity Handout 1: "Personality Patterns"
Lead feedback discussion		

Evaluation: Group writes three statements refuting the myths.

LECTURE OUTLINE 3A:
RECENT FINDINGS ON PSYCHOLOGICAL ASPECTS OF AGING

I. Intelligence
   A. Questions of validity in cross-sectional testing of intelligence and longitudinal
   B. Recognition of complexity of testing
   C. Recognition of differences in testing older adults
      1. Cohort
      2. Education level
      3. Motivation
      4. Practice
      5. Speed
   D. Intelligence plateau during the life span
   E. Increase in intelligence over the life span on some measures
   F. Terminal drop

II. Learning
   A. Differences between learning styles of adults and children
      1. Motivation, purpose
      2. Race, response time
      3. Practice

III. Memory
   A. In normal aging: adequate for most tasks of daily life
   B. Value of exercise
   C. Use of memory aids (e.g., imagery)
   D. Memory loss as indicator of health problem

LECTURE OUTLINE 3B: PATHOLOGICAL CONDITIONS IN PSYCHOLOGICAL AGING

I.   Prevalence of pathological conditions
   A.   Estimated at 60% for population over 65
   B.   Percentage rises with age
II. Importance of careful diagnosis
   A.   Irreversible brain disorders (dementias of the Alzheimer type) have frequently been confused with reversible conditions such as delirium (temporary confusion), depression, physical illness
   B.   Dementia and depression may exhibit similar but different symptoms
   C.   Complete personal social medical history must be taken
   D.   Alzheimer's disease can only be accurately diagnosed by autopsy
   E.   Misdiagnosing depression or delirium as dementia may result in no treatment for a treatable condition
III. Types of organic disorders (also called dementias or senile/dementia)
   A.   Alzheimer's disease
      1.   Most debilitating, progressive
      2.   Producing family stress
   B.   Parkinson's disease
   C.   Creutzfeld-Jakob disease
   D.   Pick's disease
   E.   Multi-infarct (ministroke)
IV. General symptoms of pathological states
   A.   Impairment of memory
   B.   Impairment of judgment, reasoning skill
   C.   Disorientation
   D.   Inappropriate behaviors
   E.   Inattention to personal care
   F.   Apathy
   G.   Irritability
V.   Possible causes of temporary confusion
   A.   Infection
   B.   Heart, liver disease
   C.   Malnutrition
   D.   Drug intoxication
   E.   Dehydration
   F.   Surgery, anesthesia
   G.   Isolation
   H.   Sudden environmental change
VI. Depression
   A.   Major depressive reaction
   B.   Manic-depressive illness
   C.   Potential for recovery
   D.   Possible confusion in diagnosis with dementia

PERSONALITY PATTERNS

1. Divide into pairs:
    a. Each person thinks of someone he/she has known into old age and describes that person to his/her partner. Talk about personality traits, life-style, mental health, activities.
    b. After each partner has described a person, list characteristics common to both and unique characteristics of each. Which might be due to age and which represent long-term traits?
    c. Are they more alike or more different?
2. a. Whole group: Use photo set of well-known older people who make or made real contributions to society. Identify each and his/her contribution.
    b. Each person thinks of someone over 65 who is making real contributions to society today. Going round robin, give each person time to briefly describe his/her person.
3. What do you think you'll be like at age 70? What personality traits will be strong? What life-style do you expect to have? What kinds of activities will you be doing? What will be your greatest joys? Write several paragraphs describing yourself at age 70.

LESSON PLAN, SESSION 4: SOCIAL ASPECTS OF NORMAL AGING

Competencies: I (C-3): Trainees will know and be able to discuss social dimensions of aging

II (A): Trainees will be able to recognize and refute myths about aging persons

Objectives: I (I): Trainees will be able to discuss role loss and role assignment as these apply to the older population

I (J): Trainees will be able to list five possible roles in later life

Instructor	Trainee	Materials
Distribute Activity Handout 1: "Society's Signals"	Complete handout	Activity Handout 1: "Society's Signals"
Introduce concept of social aging (Lecture Outline 4.I)	Take notes or underline text	Primary text, Chapter 2
Lead discussion on the roles allocated to older persons	Contribute ideas	
Present concept of loss and later life (Lecture Outline 4.II)		Primary text, Chapter 2
Distribute and explain Activity Handout 2: "Values and Losses"; lead feed-back discussion	Follow instructions of Activity Handout 2: "Values and Losses"; compare notes	Activity Handout 2: "Values and Losses"
Lead class to compile list of problems faced by older adults that reflect our society's view toward aging on chalkboard or flipchart		Chalkboard or flipchart
Present information about social aging as interpretation/adaption (Lecture Outline 4.III)	Take notes or underline text	Primary text, Chapter 2
Present concept of social network and its significance in successful aging	Take notes or underline text	Primary text, Chapter 2
Distribute Activity Handout 3: "Social Network"	Draw social network	Activity Handout 3: "Social Network"
Lead feedback discussion		

Evaluation: Review responses on Activity Handout 1: "Society's Signals" to see if attitudes have changed.

LECTURE OUTLINE 4: SOCIAL AGING

I. Social aging refers to the roles assigned by society to aging individuals, and the behaviors regarded as appropriate for their age
   A. Some gerontologists project an "age-irrelevant" society

II. Older people respond in different ways to role loss and role assignments
   A. Society assigns roles
      1. Retiree
      2. "Old"
      3. Nonproductive
      4. Sick, senile
   B. Individuals can passively accept negative role assignment, act out myths (see Chapter 2, Figure 2.2)
   C. Individuals can reject such role assignments and
      1. Find new innovative roles
      2. Become useful
      3. Do not permit "labeling"

III. Successful aging is in large part successful adaptation to change
   A. Coping style and way of adapting in the earlier stages of life is an important antecedent to successful adaptation in later life
   B. Poor coping skills in early life may lead to difficulties in dealing with change in later life
   C. Changes may come rapidly in later life (i.e., several in close succession)
   D. Replacement of lost roles by new ones, sought out or created, represents successful adaptation to aging

SOCIETY'S SIGNALS

We often expect people to behave in certain ways when they reach a particular age. At what age, if at all, should a person:

(write in age)

1. Begin to work? _____
2. Marry? _____
3. Have children? _____
4. Buy a house? _____
5. Graduate from college? _____
6. Change careers? _____
7. Retire? _____
8. Slow down? _____

How do you feel about a person age 70 who:

(check appropriate response)

1. Marries? ____ OK ____ NOT OK
2. Graduates from college? ____ OK ____ NOT OK
3. Begins to work? ____ OK ____ NOT OK
4. Changes careers? ____ OK ____ NOT OK
5. Does not retire? ____ OK ____ NOT OK
6. Fathers a baby? ____ OK ____ NOT OK

Discuss (in small groups): Is our society in the process of becoming "age irrelevant"?

VALUES AND LOSSES

1. Instructor provides 10 small cards or pieces of paper for each trainee.
2. Trainees write on each card the name of person, possession, freedom, etc. which he/she presently enjoys and on which he/she places a *high value*.
3. Trainees then organize cards in terms of which could be most easily given up first, second, third, and so forth.
4. Trainees compare notes.

SOCIAL NETWORK

1. Diagram or draw your current social network. (Invent the pattern, e.g., a tree, circles, web)
2. Draw or diagram the social network of very old person, or a developmentally disabled person.
3. Compare and evaluate these for overall strength.

LESSON PLAN, SESSION 5: LIVING ARRANGEMENTS

Competency: I (E): Trainees will know and be able to discuss options in living arrangements for older adults
Objective: I (K): Trainees will be able to list six options for living arrangements during the later years

Instructor	Trainee	Materials
List on chalkboard or flipchart all options in living arrangements available to the older population	Make own list Discuss complete list	Chalkboard or flipchart
Lead discussion about most preferred and least preferred living arrangements? Why?	Discuss	
Present information on family proximity, sex differences, and rural/urban differences in living arrangements (Lecture Outline 5)	Take notes or underline text	Primary text, Chapter 3

Evaluation: Each trainee makes a continuum line with "independent" at one end and "dependent" at the other. List the six options on the line.

LECTURE OUTLINE 5: LIVING ARRANGEMENTS

I. Older adults are not abandoned by families
    A. Most live within 30 minutes to 1 hour of a close relative
    B. Most are in contact by phone or mail if separated by many miles
    C. Most do not prefer to live with family
    D. Most will live with family if necessary
    E. Families make a significant effort to help
    F. Families are major support system to older relatives
II. There are significant differences in living arrangements of the elderly
    A. Over three fourths of older men live with a spouse
    B. Almost half of older women live alone
    C. The great majority of nursing home residents are women

LESSON PLAN, SESSION 6: ECONOMIC AND WORK CHANGES

Competency: I (F): Trainees will know and be able to discuss income and work changes with aging
Objective: I (L): Trainees will be able to illustrate by graph drawing changes in income that occur with retirement

Instructor	Trainee	Materials
Present income graph (Primary text, Chapter 3, Figure 3.1)		Transparency or blow-up of Figure 3.1
Present facts about retirement (Lecture Outline 6.I–II)	Take notes or underline text	Primary text, Chapter 3
Reality test: Direct group to think of/ list older persons they know who have/ have not retired. What are the reasons for their choice?	List Discuss	
Distribute and explain Activity Handout 1: "It's a Great Retirement"	Complete story problem in activity handout	Activity Handout 1: "It's a Great Retirement"
Present information about economic trends affecting older people (Lecture Outline 6.III)	Take notes or underline text	Primary text, Chapter 3
Refer to graphs in primary text, Section I	Give examples	
Lead discussion		

Evaluation: Group writes three or four summary statements about economic condition of older adults.

LECTURE OUTLINE 6: RETIREMENT

I.   Mandatory retirement age was changed from 65 to 70 in 1978 and in 1986 was elimi-
     nated altogether except for a few categories
     A.   Rate of retirement for men has increased greatly since 1900
          1.   Because of Social Security
          2.   Because of private pension plans
          3.   Because of early retirement incentives
          4.   About 18% of older men currently remain in work force
     B.   The number of older women in the work force has remained fairly stable over the
          years, but is increasing at present
II. Retirement often brings financial change and difficulty
     A.   Average reduction in income is about 40%
     B.   Changes in Medicare have put more of the cost of medical expenses upon the
          older person
     C.   According to current data, one out of seven persons over 65 now lives in poverty
          1.   When those in "near poverty" are included it is about 21%
          2.   The majority are women
          3.   Blacks/Hispanics are overrepresented in the elderly poor
III. Retirement and work trends of the future
     A.   Many older people indicate that they would like to continue to work in some
          capacity
          1.   Many choose to work to increase income
          2.   Many wish to work to stay useful
          3.   Many feel "young" enough to continue work
          4.   Many do not want to leave the mainstream
     B.   Need for older workers may increase
     C.   Recent recessions and technological changes have displaced many middle-aged
          workers
          1.   Some are being retrained through special programs in business, industry,
               community
          2.   Others fall through the cracks

IT'S A GREAT RETIREMENT

You are a 75-year-old widow living alone on a fixed income from a pension plan your husband had, plus Social Security as a widow. Your yearly income is $6,000.

How much weekly? _____

How much monthly? _____

Make a budget to meet your needs:

Apartment rent _____

Utilities _____

Health care _____

Food _____

Transportation _____

Donations _____

Recreation _____

Emergencies _____

How much is left over? _____

Discuss the quality of life on that income. How might one be able to economize?

LESSON PLAN, SESSION 7: LEISURE, RECREATION, AND COMMUNITY SERVICES

Competencies: I (G): Trainees will know and be able to discuss leisure and recreational preferences of older persons
I (H): Trainees will know and be able to discuss community services provided by the Older Americans Act and by various organizations/agencies
II (B): Trainees will be able to locate information about aging
II (C): Trainees will be able to identify community services that can be accessed by older adults

Objectives: I (M): Trainees will be able to define the Older Americans Act
I (N): Trainees will be able to list eight community services specifically provided for older adults
I (O): Trainees will be able to describe the concept of formal and informal support systems

Instructor	Trainee	Materials
Review concepts from the film *Aging*; explain diversity of older people in terms of varied interests, abilities, experiences, motivation, etc. (Lecture Outline 7A)	Discuss, take notes	Primary text, Chapter 3
Illustrate diversity by listing interests of trainees on chalkboard or flipchart	Contribute to list	Chalkboard or flipchart
Discuss which interests would be dropped or altered by the aging process	Discuss	
Present case histories, or draw from class experience of older persons who have acquired *new* leisure interests, activities, or careers; emphasize retirement as opportunity	Discuss	Resource: McLeish: *The Challenge of Aging* (see Additional Readings, Section I, primary text)
Present information about the Older Americans Act and other community services for older adults (Lecture Outline 7B)	Take notes or underline text	Primary text, Chapter 4
Review list of community services (Primary text, Chapter 4, Table 4.2)		Transparency or blow-up of Table 4.2

Evaluation: Generate a list of local recreational and community services for older adults.

LECTURE OUTLINE 7A: LEISURE AND RECREATION

I. Individuals choose individual life-styles in later life
    A. These frequently reflect earlier interests and skills
    B. The typical life-style usually includes activity or affiliation of some kind
        1. Activity is thought to promote well-being
        2. Equates with high life satisfaction
    C. Disengagement (the rocking chair approach) is chosen by a small percentage
        1. It also equates with high life satisfaction as a deliberately chosen life-style
    D. Low income is not in itself a deterrent to pursuit of leisure and recreational activities in later life
        1. Senior centers offer many opportunities at little cost
        2. Some form of senior transportation is available in most communities
    E. Physical changes may affect choices and/or cause adjustments in recreation and leisure pursuits
        1. Less energy
        2. Sensory changes
        3. Decreased mobility
II. There is a broad range of options for recreational and leisure time activities
    A. Travel
    B. Volunteer and part-time work
        1. At least 800,000 retired senior volunteers are involved annually
        2. Church activities
        3. Advocacy for peace and other causes
        4. Peace Corps, Vista
    C. Lifetime learning
        1. Continuing education
        2. Informal learning opportunities
        3. Elderhostel
    D. Hobbies
    E. Physical exercise
        1. Senior Olympics

LECTURE OUTLINE 7B: THE OLDER AMERICANS ACT

I.   History of the Older Americans Act
     A.   Passed by Congress, 1965
     B.   Based on recommendations of White House Conference on Aging in 1961
     C.   Amended in major ways over the years
     D.   Reauthorized every 3 years to present
     E.   Originally authorized funds for administration and research and development

II. Major provisions at present
     A.   Organized under six titles
         1. Separately funded
     B.   Administration is through a national network
         1. Administration on Aging (National)
         2. State departments or commissions
         3. Local area agencies on aging
             a. Geographically contiguous throughout the country
             b. Divisions based upon numbers of persons over age 60
     C.   Title III provides for a wide variety of services without eligibility guidelines other than age
         1. Nutrition
         2. Socialization
         3. Assessment
         4. Transportation
         5. Information and referral
         6. Outreach
         7. Homemaker and chore service
         8. Legal aid
         9. Long-term care ombudsman
     D.   Training and research are funded under Title IV
     E.   An older worker program with eligibility guidelines comprises Title V
     F.   Title VI describes rights of Native Americans

AUDIOVISUAL RESOURCES

Aging (21 min.), color, 1973, H-A,S; (Educational Psychology Series): Examines some popular, yet commonly mistaken, attitudes toward the aged and their place in society. Discusses two major theories on the aged—the Activity Theory and the Disengagement Theory—and the research being done by Bernice Neugarten, Robert Havighurst, and Sheldon Tobin, of the University of Chicago. Discussion guide.

Antonia: A Portrait of the Woman (58 min.), color, 1974, J-A; 2 reels: Presents a portrait of Antonia Brico, who in the 1930s, established an international reputation as an accomplished orchestra conductor. Today, she teaches conducting and piano in Denver, and leads the Brico Symphony, a community orchestra which she founded. Study guide.

Because Somebody Cares (27 min.), color, 1979, J-A: A community program where volunteers visit shut-in senior citizens. They help with simple tasks or provide a friendly exchange. Younger participants are particularly enthusiastic about their elderly friends.

Detour (13 min.), color, 1977, J-C,A: Eighty-three-year-old Catherine Hamilton lives in a hospital bed, retreating into those memories she holds most dear. She is ready for her death but others are in control of her destiny. Small wonder that she stubbornly fights in her own behalf. Discussion guide.

Everybody Rides the Carousel, Pt. 3 (24 min.), color, 1976, H-A: Faith and John Hubley's animated interpretation of the eight stages of life outlined in the works of psychologist Erik Erikson. The last two stages of life are adulthood and old age. Adulthood is the longest ride, varying between creation and stagnation. In old age, people must face the fact of aging and inevitable death. Discussion guide.

Everybody Rides the Carousel: In Later Years (8 min.), color, 1978, H-A: Highly amusing animation by Faith Hubley showing that some people definitely age more gracefully than others. Contrasts two elderly couples, one visiting a cafeteria and the other entertaining children for trick-or-treat.

Growing Old: Something to Live for (14 min.), color, 1977, C,A: Focuses on successful adaptations to growing old: working persons over 65 and happily retired people living as they wish in familiar neighborhoods. Points out that the elderly are an emerging minority of individuals, not stereotypes. Guide.

Hattie (9 min.), B & W, 1975, H-A: Interviews with a 76-year-old woman who contrasts her active past life with her present one, which is full of loneliness and financial insecurity. Discussion guide.

Maggie Kuhn: Wrinkled Radical (27 min.), color, 1975, H-A: Profiles Gray Panthers leader Maggie Kuhn and her efforts in protecting the rights of the elderly. Shows her being interviewed in her home by Studs Terkel, working in the Panthers' Philadelphia offices, and speaking with groups about discrimination against the aged.

Raisin Wine (12 min.), color, A: Presents a portrait and brief biographical sketch of Harry Oliver, motion picture art director and hermit, now a member of the Motion Picture Company Home. He reminisces about his life and records his feelings on aging.

Rose by Any Other Name: About Sexuality and Aging (15 min.), color, 1977, H-A,S: A trigger film dramatizing the needs of older people for privacy and love. Designed to help in exploring societal and institutional attitudes toward the elderly and their sexual needs. Discussion guide.

Shopping Bag Lady (21 min.), color, 1975, J-A: A series of encounters between an elderly transient woman and a group of teenaged girls who harass her is used to illustrate the desperate need for greater compassion and human understanding. Discussion guide.

Trigger Films on Aging (14 min.), color, 1971, A: A discussion film on problems of the aged. Presents 5 vignettes, each establishing a problem situation in the life of an elderly person, which builds to an emotional climax and abruptly ends.

What Do You See, Nurse? (12 min.), color, 1980, J-A: Poetic pleading of a nursing home resident to disregard the infirmities of her age and truly see her—not as a crabby old woman who dribbles her food, but as someone who has lived fully and loved deeply. Discussion guide.

Wild Goose (18 min.), B & W, 1975, H-A: Look at one elderly man's rebellion against life in a convalescent home as he antagonizes other residents and chases nurses in his wheelchair. Depicts the man's struggle against conformity.

Viewing Level Codes: A = Adult Education & General Use; C = Junior College, University; H = High School (Grades 10–12); J = Junior High (Grades 7–9); S = Special Education.

Nature and Needs of Elderly Persons with Mental Retardation/ Developmental Disabilities

COMPETENCIES

I. Knowledge: Trainees will know and be able to discuss accurately
  A. The definition of developmental disabilities and of mental retardation and the terms used in those definitions
  B. The distinctions between mild, moderate, severe, and profound retardation
  C. The characteristics of older adults with developmental disabilities as found in research studies in terms of
    1. Cognitive development
    2. Social competence
    3. Physical condition
    4. Living arrangements and economic status
    5. Leisure, recreation, and community service utilization
       a. Community access implementation model
  D. Concepts related to services for people with developmental disabilities
    1. Individualized
    2. Interdisciplinary
    3. Coordinated
  E. Terminology used in the field, including
    1. Generic/special
    2. Habilitation
    3. Sheltered employment
  F. Agencies that provide services to persons with developmental disabilities
    1. State agencies
    2. Nonpublic agencies
    3. Advocacy and information organizations
    4. Recreation/leisure
    5. Service coordination
  G. Types of community residential alternatives and their services, including:
    1. Individual residential services
    2. Group residential services
  H. Habilitation/work activities
    1. Work and related training
       a. Sheltered employment

    b. Competitive employment
    c. Supported employment
   2. Training in self-help, daily living, social and recreational skills
   3. Adult activity programs
   4. Retirement or older client programs
  I. Support services
   1. Physical health services
   2. Occupational therapy, physical therapy, psychology, mental health
   3. Transportation
  J. Where to find information about financial support, including Social Security, Bureau of Vocational Rehabilitation
  K. Formal and informal support networks
   1. Advocacy
   2. Guardianship
   3. Family support services
   4. Respite care
   5. Self-help mutual support groups
II. Skills: Trainees will be able to
  A. Understand the needs of developmentally disabled individuals and know which agencies should be able to meet those needs

OBJECTIVES

 I. Knowledge: Trainees will be able to
  A. Know the essential elements of the definition of developmental disabilities
   1. Attributable to mental or physical impairment
   2. Manifested before age 22
   3. Likely to continue indefinitely
   4. Resulting in substantial functional limitations in three or more areas of major life activity
   5. Requiring special services
  B. When given a list of the areas of major life activity, define and give examples of each area
  C. List or select from choices the three essential elements of the AAMD definition of mental retardation
   1. Significantly subaverage general intellectual functioning
   2. Concurrent with deficits in adaptive behavior
   3. Manifested in the developmental period
  D. When given the three elements of the AAMD definition, define each as it relates to retardation
  E. Distinguish between the levels of retardation (mild, moderate, severe, and profound) by writing at least three characteristics of each level or selecting them from a list
  F. State briefly the major findings of the ACCESS study and other research presented about older adults with mental retardation/developmental disabilities in the areas of
   1. Psychological and cognitive development
   2. Social competence
   3. Physical condition

G.   Using the training materials, discuss the living arrangements and economic status of these older adults and compare them to those of average peers

H.   State briefly the major findings of the ACCESS study and other research presented about older adults with mental retardation/developmental disabilities with regard to leisure, recreation, and community services utilization

I.   Describe the Kennedy Companion model for assisting older adults with MR/DD to access community recreational and support services

J.   List at least five generic and five special services that could be utilized by non-retarded developmentally disabled individuals

K.   Given a list of residential options and a number of possible services or characteristics, match the services to the type of residential option

L.   Write a paragraph distinguishing between habilitation and work activities and discussing the importance of each

M.   List and describe modifications in programming for older clients of retirement age

N.   Given the words "advocacy," "guardianship," and "family support services," match services to providers

O.   Describe how a developmentally disabled person might be assisted to live in the community using only support services

II.   Skill: Trainees will be able to

A.   Given four descriptions of persons with handicaps, choose those who are developmentally disabled

B.   Verbally or in a written paragraph discuss the differences in service needs of nonretarded persons with developmental disabilities in terms of duration, variety of needs, need to be with nonretarded peers

III.   Attitude: Trainees will

A.   Use proper terminology when referring to *persons who have disabilities* rather than "the retarded" or "retarded people"

LESSON PLAN, SESSION 1: DEFINITIONS

Competencies: I (A): Trainees will know and be able to discuss the definitions of developmental disabilities and of mental retardation and the terms used in those definitions

    I (B): Trainees will know and be able to discuss the distinctions between mild, moderate, severe, and profound retardation

Objectives: I (A): Trainees will know the essential elements of the definition of developmental disabilities

    I (B): When given a list of the areas of major life activities, trainees will define and give examples of each area

    I (C): Trainees will list or select from choices the three essential elements of the AAMD definition of mental retardation

    I (D): When given the three elements of the AAMD definition, trainees will be able to define each as it relates to retardation

    I (E): Trainees will distinguish between the levels of retardation (mild, moderate, severe, and profound) by writing at least three characteristics of each level or selecting them from a list

Instructor	Trainee	Materials
Discuss definition of developmental disability (Lecture Outline 1.I, 1.II)	Take notes or underline text; if desired, read the definition and explanation of developmental disabilities in Chapter 2 of the primary text	Primary text, Chapter 5
Distribute Activity Handout 1: "Decisions About Developmental Disabilities"	With other members of your group, decide whether each case presented is eligible for services as a person who is Substantially Developmentally Disabled (SDD)	Activity Handout 1: "Decisions about Developmental Disabilities"

Discuss definition of mental retardation (Lecture Outline 1.III, 1.IV)		Primary text, Chapter 5
Distribute and discuss Handout 1: "Typical Life Experiences of Older Developmentally Disabled People"		Handout 1: "Typical Life Experiences of Older Developmentally Disabled People"
Activity: Divide class into four groups; assign each group one level of retardation to write a "composite person"	Each group reads the description in the book, then composes a paragraph describing a composite person at that level of retardation	Paper and pens

Evaluation: Have class list essential components of DD and MR definitions

LECTURE OUTLINE 1:
DEVELOPMENTAL DISABILITIES/MENTAL RETARDATION DEFINITIONS

I. Five elements of the federal definition of developmental disability
    A. Attributable to mental or physical impairment or combination of mental and physical impairments (e.g., mental retardation, spina bifida, cerebral palsy with retardation)
    B. Manifested before the person attains age 22
        1. Developmental period
            a. Learning depending upon interaction with environment (e.g., child with CP can't get around to interact)
            b. More complex learning dependent on previous learning experience (e.g., reading depends on knowing names of things in environment)
        2. Service needs
            a. Children with DD in school until age 22
            b. MR/DD system for those disabled in developmental period; Bureau of Vocational Rehabilitation, Goodwill, United Cerebral Palsy, others for those who become disabled in later life
    C. Is likely to continue indefinitely
        1. Need for long-term supports
        2. Temporary disabilities have temporary effects (e.g., child with CP will never "recover," needs lifelong services; child in auto accident who is in hospital for 6 months can make up schoolwork)
    D. Results in substantial functional/limitations in three or more areas of major life activity
        1. Functional definition
            a. Many people with disabilities from their developmental period are able to live normal lives (e.g., Thomas Edison, Stevie Wonder)
            b. Definition is for purpose of deciding eligibility for services; those most needful of help to be chosen
            c. Limitation of resources makes it necessary to serve only those most in need; others also have needs, but there isn't enough for all
    E. Reflects the person's needs for combination and sequence of special, interdisciplinary, or generic care, treatment or other services that are lifelong or of extended duration and are individually planned and coordinated
        1. No assumption of total care requiring institutional placement
            a. Can be in-and-out care
            b. Can use only parts of the system (OT/PT, speech)
II. Areas of major life activities
    A. Self-care—examples: eating, drinking, dressing, toileting, bathing, grooming
    B. Receptive and expressive language—ability to understand words, symbols, messages from others (receptive language); ability to communicate wants, needs, ideas verbally or by sign or symbol (expressive language)
    C. Learning—the ability to benefit from experience, to add new information; usually indicated by IQ range
    D. Mobility—the ability to move about the environment; refers to both ambulation and finding locations
    E. Self-direction—the ability to behave appropriately without attracting attention to oneself

    F.   Capacity for independent living—ability to live independently and manage one's own affairs

    G. Economic self-sufficiency—ability to keep and hold a job and to manage money

III. Definition of mental retardation—three elements (credit to AAMD)

    A. Significantly subaverage general intellectual functioning

       1. (draw on board or use chart) Show bell curve, indicate where three standard deviations below mean is and discuss implications

       2. Discuss low incidence relative to the curve

    B. Existing concurrently with deficits in adaptive behavior

       1. Provision put in to prevent minorities from being labeled and inappropriately placed (relates to functional definition of DD)

       2. Low adaptive behavior alone doesn't qualify

    C. Manifested in the developmental period

       1. Same as DD definition

       2. Results in learning deficits

IV. Definitions of key words (definitions are found in the primary text)

    A. General intellectual functioning

    B. Significantly subaverage general intellectual functioning

    C. Adaptive behavior

    D. Developmental period

    E. Mental retardation

DECISIONS ABOUT DEVELOPMENTAL DISABILITIES

Decide whether each of these individuals is developmentally disabled under the federal definition. Explain why the person is or isn't eligible for services.

John has had cerebral palsy since birth. He is in a wheelchair all day from the time he gets up, dresses, eats, gets in his car, and goes to work until he comes home and gets ready for bed. He will always have this disability.

_____

_____

_____

Joe is a paraplegic. He broke his neck diving at a rock quarry while on an outing with his wife and children. He has difficulty talking, cannot be understood by others, cannot move independently, and must have all of his body needs taken care of by others. He is totally dependent.

_____

_____

_____

Jane has severe epilepsy which first appeared in high school. Her seizures are not controlled well enough for her to hold a job or get a driver's license. She has been unable to live alone because of the danger of injury during seizures.

_____

_____

_____

Lou was in a special education class in school. She reads very poorly and with many mistakes. She can handle money well enough to make small purchases, but can't budget or manage a paycheck. She has held about 15 entry-level jobs since high school, none for more than a week. She lost these jobs because of her poor judgment and inability to get along with her employers or co-workers.

_____

_____

_____

TYPICAL LIFE EXPERIENCES OF
OLDER DEVELOPMENTALLY DISABLED PEOPLE

People who have developmental disabilities have many more problems than the actual disabilities. The effects of their handicap are compounded by the reactions of others, their own diminished experience, and personal perceptions of being devalued members of society.

From earliest childhood those who have physical and/or mental impairments are seen as "different" by others. Nonhandicapped people may stare or make fun of them. Some people are oversympathetic or too helpful. Others feel embarrassed and simply avoid looking at or talking to people with disabilities. When they are young, people with developmental disabilities rarely play with other children. As they get older, there are few contacts with others, especially those who are "normal." They experience rejection over and over again until they come to expect it. People who expect to be rejected have great difficulty meeting others. They are defeated in social contacts before they start, so their behavior is often inappropriate.

Society separates itself from those considered deviant in several ways. One way is to actually bring them all together in a remote setting. Institutions have served this purpose for many years. Mentally retarded persons have been removed from their homes and communities and placed with others "like themselves." In such settings they lose all control of their lives and learn to become dependent on others. Every activity of their day is regulated by the institutional staff; the residents do not learn to make decisions about their own lives.

Residents of institutions live, eat, and work with assigned groups. Until recently there was little training for them. In Ohio until the 1960s, institutions were run as farms with the work done by residents. Old-timers at Apple Creek remember working in its orchards and fields or caring for livestock. The farm products were used to feed residents of all the state's institutions. The farm jobs paid little or nothing but there was a positive side in that the workers engaged in healthy outdoor activity and performed a useful function. Their lives had some meaning. In the 1960s the so-called "peonage" laws put an end to exploitation of workers' labor and most residents were returned to lives of idleness or limited activities.

Until recently, when families chose to keep their disabled relative at home, the full burden of training and socialization fell on them. Public schools excluded children with IQs below 50 until the late 1970s. Most disabled children and adults just stayed at home. Their contacts were limited to family and family friends. Their experiences were only those that could be provided by the family. Many of them were aware that they were a source of anguish to their loved ones and that their care was a constant problem.

Until the advent of sheltered workshops, employment was nonexistent for these people. Some worked around their homes or family farms. Many were dependent upon Social Security or SSI for financial support. Even with the pay earned on a prorated basis in a sheltered workshop, the income of most older retarded persons is at the poverty level.

Experiences of disabled people are limited both by their condition and by society's provisions for them. It is difficult to develop personal relationships when there are few opportunities for contacts with others; and the contacts that occur are usually characterized by anxiety about rejection. Retarded people are limited in their ability to go places by themselves; there is almost always a caregiver with them. It is hard to develop self-confidence when one's own judgment can't be trusted, and when decisions are always made by others. Developmentally disabled persons rarely have been encouraged to be interested in members of the opposite sex. Their emotional lives were expected to remain on a child's level, limited to "liking" someone. Normal sexual expression has been discouraged or prohibited. Love and marriage were not for them.

Small wonder, then, that people who are devalued and impoverished in all aspects of life come to dislike themselves. The cumulative effect of their life experiences constantly makes them aware of their incompetence and dependence on others. It would be hard for the strongest ego to withstand so many negative messages.

Marion Stroud, Ph.D.

Discussion Questions

1. What emotions are aroused by rejection? How do people act when they expect to be rejected?
2. How are developmentally disabled people deprived of learning experiences when they are kept separate from the mainstream of society?
3. What benefits might both groups expect from more contact and knowledge of each other?

LESSON PLAN, SESSION 2: PSYCHOLOGICAL AND COGNITIVE CHARACTERISTICS

Competency: I (C-1): Trainees will know and be able to discuss the cognitive development characteristics of older adults with MR/DD as found in research studies

Objective: I (F-1): Trainees will be able to state briefly the major findings of the ACCESS study and other research presented about older adults with MR/DD in terms of psychological and cognitive development

Instructor	Trainee	Materials
Discuss psychological and cognitive characteristics of older adults with MR/DD (Lecture Outline 2)	Take notes or underline text	Primary text, Chapter 6; transparencies or blow-ups of Tables 6.1 and 6.2
Select an activity from Activity 1: "Remembering Past Lives"	Participate in the activity	Leader's instructions, Activity 1: "Remembering Past Lives"; pictures of famous older people

Evaluation: Have each participant write or state the major findings about cognitive development from ACCESS research study

LECTURE OUTLINE 2:
PSYCHOLOGICAL AND COGNITIVE CHARACTERISTICS OF ACCESS STUDY SUBJECTS

I.   Demographics (Tables 6.1, p. 52, primary text)
   A.   Intelligence range
      1.   30% were in the severe/profound range
      2.   44% were in the moderate range
      3.   27% measured either mild or normal—they are called SDD (substantially developmentally disabled) because they have become functionally retarded as a result of institutionalization or deprivation of life experience

II. Learning
   A.   Schooling
      1.   Few attended school at all—common belief that retarded people were not educable
      2.   Those who attended school were usually asked to leave at about second grade because of failure to read
   B.   Functional academic skills (Table 6.2, p. 53, primary text)
      1.   Reading—most are nonreaders; some know "survival" words: "stop," "men," "exit," etc.
      2.   Writing—most can write name only
      3.   Money—few can use functionally; some use coins in vending machines; make purchases with total supervision
      4.   Time—few can tell time more than to hour; calendar used only with extensive assistance

III. Communication (Table 6.2, p. 53, primary text)
   A.   Receptive language
      1.   About two thirds understood most spoken communication
      2.   The rest respond either to simple requests or to their names
   B.   Expressive language
      1.   Overall communication level nearly normal for about two thirds
      2.   85% use speech to communicate
      3.   Content of talk simple and brief
   C.   Conversation skills
      1.   Most lack ability to carry on a conversation
      2.   Need to learn small-talk skills

IV. Summary
   A.   These subjects of the ACCESS study were young at a time when school was not encouraged for them; most either didn't attend at all or left school by request when they failed to learn to read, at about second grade; they are essentially nonreaders, nonwriters, and have only a few skills with money and time
   B.   Their communication is largely using spoken words, and the content is sparse and simply spoken; they understand most of what is said to them if it is said in simple form

REMEMBERING PAST LIVES (Leader's Instructions)

Purpose

1. To remember a person known over many years from youth to older age
2. To discover whether psychological traits change or persist
3. To acknowledge that older people make real contributions to society
4. To make predictions about self in older age

Activities

1. a. Have trainees form pairs for sharing. Ask each person to remember someone he/she has known for a long time, such as a grandparent or older friend. Each partner should talk about the remembered persons' personality traits, life-style, mental health, activities, and preferences.
   b. Have partners list the characteristics the remembered people had in common, and the unique characteristics of each. Partners should decide which might be due to age and which seem to be long-term traits.
   c. Ask partners to discuss whether the persons are more alike or more different.
2. Have trainees look at pictures of famous older people who are making or have made real contributions to society in their old age. Ask them to identify each and discuss what he/she did, and how maturity influenced their contributions.
3. Have each person tell about an older person known to him/her who is making a contribution to society in some way, and describe the effects of that person's maturity on what is done.
4. Have a group discussion of the following ideas: "What do you think you will be like when you are old? What traits do you think will persist? What kinds of activities will you expect to be interested in doing? How will your personality change? What will be your greatest joys?"

Materials

1. Pictures of famous older people

LESSON PLAN, SESSION 3: SOCIAL COMPETENCE

Competency: I (C-2): Trainees will know and be able to discuss social competence characteristics of older adults with MR/DD as found in research studies

Objective: I (F-2): Trainees will be able to state briefly the major findings of the ACCESS study and other research presented about older adults with MR/DD in terms of social competence

Instructor	Trainee	Materials
Discuss social competence of older adult with MR/DD (Lecture Outline 3)	Take notes or underline text	Primary text, Chapter 6; transparencies or blow-ups of Tables 6.1, 6.3, 6.4, and 6.5
Select an activity from Activity 1: "Love is a Many-Splendored Thing"; *or* distribute any of the Activity Handouts for Session 4, Section I, but discuss with reference to DD adults	Participate in activity	Leader's instructions: Activity 1: "Love Is a Many-Splendored Thing"; paper and pencils; copies of Activity Handouts from Session 4, Section I as needed

Evaluation: Evaluate learning from responses to activities

LECTURE OUTLINE 3: SOCIAL COMPETENCE OF ACCESS STUDY SUBJECTS

I.   Personal social competence
    A.   Adaptive behavior (Table 2.1, p. 52, primary text)
        1.   Most were in the mild or moderate range
        2.   Adaptive behavior tended to be lower than IQ range, probably as a result of being either institutionalized or deprived of life experiences
    B.   Appearance
        1.   Most appeared to look normal for their age and work
        2.   Clothing was generally neat, clean, and appropriate
        3.   Hair and grooming was similar to others of same age
        4.   Only major appearance shocker was terrible teeth
    C.   Self-care skills (Table 6.2, p. 55, primary text)
        1.   80% performed all self-care skills independently
        2.   Those who required verbal prompts, usually hand washing, shaving
II. Interaction social competence (Table 6.4, p. 55, primary text)
    A.   Interactions with other individuals
        1.   60% of interactions were usually appropriate
        2.   Inappropriate interactions included hugging, asking personal questions, and stereotyped behaviors
        3.   Tendency to be passive in all interactions
            a.   Discuss effect of institutional living on conditioning to be passive
            b.   "Those who go along, get along"
    B.   Friends, relationships were few, marriage was rare
III. Maladaptive behaviors (Table 6.5, p. 56, primary text)
        1.   Very few had any maladaptive behaviors
        2.   Those who did probably act about like other older adults
        3.   Most common maladaptive behavior was verbal aggression
            a.   Usually was name calling or cursing
            b.   Nonhandicapped people would not be noted if they did this
        4.   Other maladaptive behaviors included refusal to participate and withdrawal
            a.   Have been told what to do, where to go all their lives
            b.   Tired of being programmed and having to obey
            c.   Few or no serious destructive behaviors
IV. Summary
    A.   Most performed their self-care skills independently
    B.   They looked, acted, and dressed about like other people their age
    C.   Their interactions with others tended to be passive and limited
    D.   They have few friends and even fewer affectionate relationships
    E.   Few had even married, but many expressed the wish for someone to be close to (see Chapter 8, "Personal Perspectives," in primary text)

LOVE IS A MANY-SPLENDORED THING (Leader's Instructions)

Purpose

1. To examine the personal and social aspects of affective relationships
2. To think about one's personal social network and those of people who have developmental disabilities

Activities

1. Give each person a sheet of paper. Tell them that the activity will be personal and private. They will not be asked to share what they write. Have them list four or five kinds of affective relationships they have experienced, such as love from parents, siblings, friendships, romances, marriage, love of children, pets, neighbors, church or other organizations, work. They won't be able to do all of them but should select the most important to them to list. Ask each person to address the following questions
   a. How did each enrich your life?
   b. What were the stresses of each?
   c. Would you rate each one "plus" or "minus"?
   d. On balance, how does your affective experience come out?
2. Ask each person to draw or diagram a personal network portraying all of the people or groups who care about them—people who might be called upon for help if needed. Suggest that they can be original in the design they choose. Some may want to make a tree with branches, others may make concentric circles—whatever will show their network.

   Be aware that trainees will quickly think of family and obvious contacts; be ready to suggest less likely ones, such as people who serve us in the public or commercial sector.
3. Have the group as a whole develop a diagram of the social network of a mentally retarded and/or a developmentally disabled older adult. Have them put a dollar sign ($) beside each person (or role) in the network who is *paid* to provide the support.

Materials

1. Paper and pencil for each trainee

LESSON PLAN, SESSION 4: PHYSICAL CONDITION

Competency: I (C-3): Trainees will know and be able to discuss physical condition characteristics of older adults with MR/DD as found in research studies

Objective: I (F-3): Trainees will be able to state briefly the major findings of the ACCESS study and other research presented about older adults with MR/DD in terms of physical condition

Instructor	Trainee	Materials
Lead discussion of effects of conditions in early 20th century on physical condition of those who are now old	Participate in discussion	Primary text, Chapter 6; transparencies or blow-ups of Tables 6.1 and 6.6
Discuss physical condition of older adults with MR/DD (Lecture Outline 4)	Take notes or underline text	Leader's instructions, Activity 1, Session 2, Section I and copies of Activity Handout 1, Session 2, Section I, as needed; *or* leader's instructions, Activity 2, Session 2, Section I
Distribute Activity Handout 1: Session 2, Section I; *or* do Activity 2, Session 2, Section I, but discuss with reference to DD adults	In small groups, complete activity	
Discuss expected changes in physical condition of older persons in future	Report answers from small group activity and discuss	

Evaluation: Ask, "What did we learn?" Categories: Chronic conditions, medications, diet, use of prostheses, ambulation

LECTURE OUTLINE 4: PHYSICAL CONDITION OF ACCESS STUDY SUBJECTS

I.   Demographics (Table 6.1, p. 52, primary text)
    A.   Age: range 55–85 (about two thirds under age 65)
    B.   Sex: 54% female, 46% male
    C.   Mental retardation levels
        1.   Substantial DD (mild), 27%
        2.   Moderate retardation, 44%
        3.   Severe retardation, 24%
        4.   Profound retardation, 6%
II. Physical condition (Table 6.6, p. 57, primary text)
    A.   General health: 84% "average" (about like others their age)
    B.   Prescription medications
        1.   33% take no prescription medications
        2.   39% take one or two
        3.   28% take three or more medications (compare to average older adult)
    C.   Condition of and prosthetics use for
        1.   Vision (similar to average for age)
            a.   46% have some vision problems
            b.   Most of these have and use glasses
        2.   Hearing
            a.   35% have hearing difficulties
            b.   About 20% have and use aids
        3.   Teeth
            a.   Only 33% are relatively free of dental problems
            b.   Many have few teeth or none, many have misshapen gums and teeth in bad condition (compare to average population)
            c.   Discuss dental hygiene at the time these people were young; discuss the lack of dental hygiene or care at institutions in past
        4.   Limbs and joints
            a.   Most in fairly good condition for age
            b.   Only 10% needed canes, walkers, or wheelchairs (discuss probable early death of severely impaired in past)
    D.   Chronic conditions
        1.   Elicit "type" of condition and probable environmental aspects of most common conditions (heart disease, circulatory problems, diabetes)
            a.   Discuss change in life-style from active, outdoor life in institutions prior to "peonage laws," and sedentary, passive lives since then
            b.   Elicit "types" of conditions with low or no incidence in the study (cancer, ulcer, stroke) and discuss role of stress in these conditions
            c.   Compare stress in average lives with low-stress lives in institutions or staying at home
    E.   Diet and weight
        1.   About 60% average in weight; about 30% overweight or obese (compare to average older adults)
        2.   Discuss dietary requirements of the population: low salt, sugar free, texture modifications (similar to average population)
        3.   Concern of nutrition site operators that these people would require expensive dietary modifications not substantiated by the ACCESS study

III. Summary
   A.   The ACCESS subjects were found to compare favorably with older adults in the nonretarded population
   B.   They had fewer stress illnesses than might be expected, and most of their medical problems could be related to inactivity

LESSON PLAN, SESSION 5: LIVING ARRANGEMENTS AND ECONOMIC STATUS

Competency: I (C-4): Trainees will know and be able to discuss the living arrangements and economic status of older adults with MR/DD as found in research studies

Objective: I (G): Trainees will be able to discuss the living arrangements and economic status of these older adults and compare them to those of average peers

Instructor	Trainee	Materials
Discuss living arrangements and economic status of older adults with MR/DD (Lecture Outline 5)	Take notes or underline text	Primary text, Chapter 7
Direct Activity 1: "Living Arrangements"	Participate in activity	Leader's instructions, Activity 1: "Living Arrangements"; cost figures for various alternative residences
Distribute Activity Handout 1: "Go for Broke"	Participate in activity	Leader's instructions, Activity 2: "Economic Aspects of Aging; Activity Handout 1: "Go for Broke"; copies of Activity Handout 1, Session 6, Section I for half the participants

Evaluation: Upon completion of the activity have participants summarize the material presented.

LECTURE OUTLINE 5:
LIVING ARRANGEMENTS AND ECONOMIC STATUS OF ACCESS STUDY SUBJECTS

I.   Living arrangements
   A.   Discuss the various types of congregate living
      1.   Developmental center
      2.   Nursing home (SCF/MR)
      3.   ICF/MR and group home
      4.   Foster care
      5.   Semi-independent apartment living
      6.   Living with relatives
   B.   Discuss the living arrangements of the ACCESS subjects
      1.   The majority were in congregate settings
      2.   17% lived with various family members
      3.   11% were in semi-independent settings

II. Economic status
   A.   Income
      1.   Sources
         a.   Social Security Assistance (SSA)
         b.   Supplemental Security Income (SSI)
         c.   Veterans' or other pensions of parents
         d.   Wages from sheltered employment
      2.   Amounts—discuss and relate to poverty level
   B.   Employment
      1.   Sheltered workshop either full or part time
      2.   None in competitive employment
      3.   Many have to go on working because of need for the income

III. Summary
   A.   Most of the older adults live in congregate settings; probably this is a result of their life experiences in which they were always cared for by others and never had a chance to develop independent living skills
   B.   Their incomes place almost all of them at the poverty level

LIVING ARRANGEMENTS (Leader's Instructions)

Purpose

1. To compare alternative living arrangements for older adults in terms of advantages, disadvantages, costs, and meeting special needs of residents
2. To compare the alternative living arrangements for adults who have MR/DD in terms of advantages, disadvantages, costs, and how they meet special needs

Activities

1. List on chalkboard or chart all the alternatives for older adults listed in text. Arrange them in order from most to least independent.
2. For each one, have the trainees suggest advantages for the resident and disadvantages. It may be interesting to do the same exercise considering the families of older adults.
3. If possible, prepare a list of typical costs for each type of residence in advance. Have the trainees rank order the alternatives in terms of what they think each one costs; then rank order factually.
4. List on chalkboard or chart all the alternative living arrangements for older adults who have MR/DD presented in the text, and others if there are some. Arrange them in order from least to most restrictive.
5. In advance, get current estimated costs for each, and repeat the activity of rank ordering given in #3, above. Costs of some residences, for example, institutions, include program services. Ask trainees if these should be taken out to consider relative expense, or should be added to other settings.

Materials

1. Cost figures for the alternative residences considered

ECONOMIC ASPECTS OF AGING (Leader's Instructions)

Purpose

1. To experience vicariously the economic problems confronting older adults, both those with MR/DD and nonhandicapped older persons

Activities

1. Divide class into two groups, one to be the nonhandicapped older adults and the other to be mentally retarded employees of a sheltered workshop.
2. Give the nonhandicapped group Activity Handout 1: "It's a Great Retirement" (from Session 6, Section I) and the MR/DD group Activity Handout 1: "Go for Broke." Let them work either individually or as a group to complete the exercise. Ask them to discuss the implications of having very limited resources to meet financial needs.
3. Discuss these questions:
   a. Are basic needs provided?
   b. Are there other ways than spending money to meet these needs?
   c. What is the psychological effect of always having to be dependent on others?
4. Discuss the pros and cons of providing retirement income under Social Security for older adults who have worked in sheltered employment.

Materials

1. Enough activity sheets for each group.

GO FOR BROKE

1. *Earn big bucks:* You are an employee at a sheltered workshop. National minimum wage is $3.75 per hour. Sheltered workshop clients are paid a percentage of minimum wage equal to their percentage of performance compared to that of a normal worker.

    JOB: *Counting 20 widgets and placing in a plastic sack.*

    Time study: Nonhandicapped rate = 60/hour.

    Your rate = 15/hour.

    Your hourly pay = _____

    Your daily pay (5 hr) = _____

    Your weekly pay (5 days) = _____

2. *Spending spree:* Make up a budget for spending a week's wages (try to fit these in):

    Trip to McDonald's _____

    Bowling _____

    Toothpaste and deodorant _____

    New sleepwear _____

    Record or tape _____

    Church donation _____

    Break snacks (vending machine) _____

    Savings _____

Assumption: Person is living in a group home where basic expenses for food, shelter, and clothing are supplied

LESSON PLAN, SESSION 6: LEISURE, RECREATION, AND COMMUNITY SERVICES

Competencies: I (C-5): Trainees will know and be able to discuss leisure, recreation, and community service utilization characteristics of older adults with MR/DD as found in research studies, and will know the community access implementation model

Objectives: I (H): Trainees will be able to state briefly the major findings of the ACCESS study and other research about older adults with MR/DD with regard to leisure, recreation, and community services utilization

I (I): Trainees will describe the Kennedy Companion model for assisting older adults with MR/DD to access community recreational and support services

Instructor	Trainee	Materials
Discuss leisure activities and community service utilization of older adults with MR/DD (Lecture Outline 6)	Take notes or underline text	Primary text, Chapter 7
Distribute Activity Handout 1: "Personal Leisure/Recreation Inventory"	Participate in activity	Leader's instructions, Activity Handout 7: "Personal Leisure/Recreation Inventory and Analysis"; Activity Handout 1: "Personal Leisure/ Recreation Inventory"

Evaluation: Written or oral presentation to review lesson

LECTURE OUTLINE 6: LEISURE AND RECREATIONAL ACTIVITIES AND COMMUNITY SERVICE UTILIZATION OF ACCESS STUDY SUBJECTS

I.   Leisure activities (activities done at home) (Table 7.1, p. 66, primary text)
   A.   Most chose passive forms of leisure
      1.   Television, radio
      2.   Drinking coffee, smoking, talking to others
   B.   Some did household chores or crafts
II. Recreation (activities done away from home) (Table 7.1, p. 66, primary text)
   A.   Choices
      1.   Eating out (McDonald's)
      2.   Bowling
      3.   Shopping (see Chapter 8, primary text)
      4.   Attending fairs, sports, etc. with group
   B.   Community services utilized (Table 7.2, p. 67, primary text)
      1.   Only one person attended a senior center
      2.   No other community services were used by the group
      3.   Churches were the only agency reaching out to these people
III. Community access implementation model—The Kennedy Community Access Program (Table 7.3, p. 69, primary text)
   A.   Who participates
      1.   Older adults recommended by their program providers
      2.   Nonaffiliated older adults
      3.   Senior friends/volunteers—Kennedy Companions
   B.   How it is done
      1.   IHP team recommends to ACCESS
      2.   ACCESS assessment completed by either staff or IHP team
      3.   IHP meets (including individual) to decide whether person will become a Kennedy Senior, and if so, what special training or preparation will be done
      4.   Coordinator introduces pairs, helps in planning
   C.   Where they go
      1.   First they get acquainted, meet at residence or shop or go out for coffee together
      2.   Monthly plans made in advance to include some pure recreational activities, some attendance at senior centers—to make friends and some new experience
IV. Summary
   A.   Older adults with developmental disabilities in the ACCESS study were generally passive in their leisure activity choices; they tended to go in groups to community for recreation and shopping, with eating at McDonald's and bowling being their most common activity; they did not use community generic services
   B.   The Kennedy ACCESS model program matches older adults with MR/DD to same-age companions, either paid or volunteer; the pairs go into the community weekly to participate in recreational or learning experiences to prepare for retirement

PERSONAL LEISURE/RECREATION INVENTORY AND ANALYSIS
(Leader's Instructions)

Purpose

1. To list and analyze personal choices for leisure and recreation in terms of active and passive choices
2. To list social roles currently held and to predict future changes and effects

Activities

1. Ask each trainee to complete the Personal Leisure/Recreation Inventory. After completing it, compare active/passive ratios
2. On paper have each trainee list the social roles presently held at home, at work, and in the community. Then ask them to mark each
    a. Put a star beside those that they expect to have all of their lives
    b. Put a circle beside those that they expect will have to change as they get older
    c. Color in the circles of those that will be hard to relinquish

Materials

1. Copy of Personal Leisure/Recreation Inventory (Activity Handout 1) for each trainee

PERSONAL LEISURE/RECREATION INVENTORY

Check each activity you like to do and do as often as you can. Then for each one, circle "A" (active) if it requires you to expend energy and "P" (passive) if you can do it without much movement or interaction.

___ A P	sit or sleep		___ A P	go to movies, theater
___ A P	snack		___ A P	bowl
___ A P	chat with others		___ A P	go to party
___ A P	read books, newspapers		___ A P	attend spectator sport
___ A P	sew, crochet, knit		___ A P	play active sport
___ A P	repair, build		___ A P	shop
___ A P	cook, bake		___ A P	visit exhibits, museums
___ A P	work on car		___ A P	go to church service, social
___ A P	exercise		___ A P	attend club, lodge
___ A P	garden, do lawn work		___ A P	go to concert
___ A P	listen to radio, records		___ A P	attend club, interest group
___ A P	take a walk		___ A P	camp
___ A P	do arts or crafts		___ A P	go to fairs, carnivals
___ A P	watch television		___ A P	hear lecture, speaker
___ A P	do collecting		___ A P	visit friends
___ A P	take care of pets		___ A P	walk around mall
___ A P	grow houseplants		___ A P	play cards
___ A P	clean, rearrange		___ A P	attend classes
___ A P	do photography		___ A P	go to library
___ A P	play table games		___ A P	dance
___ A P	talk on phone		___ A P	hike
___ A P	go to restaurant			

146

LESSON PLAN, SESSION 7: SERVICES

Competencies: I (D): Trainees will know and be able to discuss concepts related to services for people with developmental disabilities

I (E): Trainees will know and be able to discuss terminology used in the field

I (F): Trainees will know and be able to discuss agencies that provide services to persons with developmental disabilities

I (G): Trainees will know and be able to discuss types of community residential alternatives and their services

Objectives: I (J): Trainees will list at least five generic and five special services that could be utilized by nonretarded developmentally disabled individuals

I (K): Given a list of residential options and a number of possible services or characteristics, trainees will match the services to the type of residential option

Instructor	Trainee	Materials
Activity: Divide into small groups; start with discussion about the similarities and differences in services needed by developmentally disabled people who *are* and who *are not* retarded; include consideration of these ideas 1. How does level of retardation affect needs for service? 2. How do physical impairments affect needs for services? 3. Is it helpful to either group to include nonretarded individuals in programs for retarded persons? Have spokesperson report ideas of each group; list on chalkboard or transparency	Participate in activity	Chalkboard or overhead projector and transparencies; if desired, copies of questions to be discussed

(continued)

147

LESSON PLAN, SESSION 7: SERVICES *(continued)*

Instructor	Trainee	Materials
Discuss concepts, terminology related to services for adults with DD; discuss agencies providing these services (Lecture Outline 7.I–7.III)	Take notes on lecture List some generic services not mentioned in the chapter Outline the section about state agencies, nonpublic agencies, and advocacy organizations, giving name and services of each Contribute ideas to discussions	Primary text, Chapter 9
Activity: Return to small groups. Review the ideas generated before the lecture and decide whether they should be modified; list the life areas in which you would expect those with DD to need assistance; again, combine the ideas of the groups on the chalkboard or transparency		
Discuss types of residential alternatives and their services (Lecture Outline 7.IV)		Primary text, Chapter 9
Have discussions related to the ideas on the chalkboard, then discuss the advantages to both the handicapped and nonhandicapped members of society from interaction in the community	Contribute ideas to discussions	

Evaluation:
Evaluate the learning using questions on Activity Handout 1: "Quiz"
	Take the quiz and correct sections answered incorrectly	Activity Handout 1: "Quiz"
		Answers in text for Questions 1 and 2
		for Question 3:
		    Developmental center—b,c,f,g
		    Group home—a,b,c,d,g
		    Foster care—a,b (some may not), e
		    Nursing home—a,b,c,f,g

LECTURE OUTLINE 7: SERVICES

I. How the needs of the developmentally disabled shape the service delivery system
  A. Needs for multiple and diverse services
    1. Medical, therapeutic
    2. Habilitation, training, vocational
    3. Residential
  B. Terms common to services for handicapped persons
    1. Interdisciplinary
    2. Individualized
    3. Coordinated
  C. Use of both generic and special services
    1. Generic services (those available to anyone who wants to use them)—includes city buses, doctors, medical clinics, post offices, stores
    2. Special services (those available only to persons who meet the specified criteria of eligibility)
    3. Some are in between; their population is specified but not limited (e.g., hospital, school)
II. State special service agencies
  A. Bureau of Vocational Rehabilitation
    1. Assessment and counseling
    2. Referrals for training and employment
    3. Funds needed for training, adaptive equipment
  B. Department of Mental Retardation/Developmental Disabilities
    1. Directs services for persons with moderate, severe, profound retardation in developmental centers
    2. Provides direction and funding for regional or local services
  C. Department of Aging
    1. Plans and sets priorities for services to elderly through area agencies on aging
    2. Directs disbursement of flow-through funds from federal and state governments to selected agencies
    3. Funds many services including nutrition programs, senior centers, homemaker services, etc.
III. Nonpublic agencies
  A. Goodwill Industries
    1. Assessment, counseling
    2. Training and sheltered employment
    3. Job placement in community employment
  B. Easter Seals
    1. Supported by donations to Easter Seals
    2. Local agencies provide a wide assortment of services, including: respite care, training, adaptive equipment, and so forth.
  C. United Cerebral Palsy (UCP)
    1. Nationwide, voluntary association of local agencies that serve people with cerebral palsy and their families
    2. Has 250 local affiliates
    3. Services can include: training, advocacy, research, sheltered employment, training of professionals, public education

D. Other advocacy and information organizations
    1. Society for Autistic Citizens
    2. Epilepsy Foundation
    3. Many other special groups involved with chronic medical conditions

IV. Residential services for developmentally disabled people who are not retarded
  A. Types of residential service options
    1. Individual
      a. Foster home
      b. Semi-independent apartment living
      c. Adoption
      d. Maintenance in family home with support
    2. Group
      a. Group homes
      b. Nursing homes
      c. Institutions other than developmental centers
  B. Characteristics of these options
    1. Foster home—individual with DD lives with a family and one or two other residents; family can receive per diem rate of reimbursement
    2. Semi-independent apartment—individual with DD lives alone or with roommate(s) with occasional assistance in meeting needs such as paying bills, shopping, cleaning, habilitation
    3. Maintenance in family home with support—in certain areas this experimental alternative to placement is being tried; support is given in home remodeling, adaptive equipment, etc.
    4. Group home—individual with DD lives in residential neighborhood in family-style home with 3–9 others; usually shares bedroom and participates in chores as if in a family
    5. Nursing home—usually like an institution in design with wards or rooms with several residents

SERVICES FOR PERSONS WITH DEVELOPMENTAL DISABILITY

1. List five generic services that could be utilized by people with developmental disabilities.

   a. _____

   b. _____

   c. _____

   d. _____

   e. _____

   List five special services that could be utilized by people with developmental disabilities.

   a. _____

   b. _____

   c. _____

   d. _____

   e. _____

2. List three services available from each of these agencies.

   a. Bureau of Vocational Rehabilitation:

   _____   _____   _____

   b. United Cerebral Palsy:

   _____   _____   _____

   c. Goodwill Industries:

   _____   _____   _____

3. Select the words that describe these residential options, and write the letters following each option.

   Developmental center _____

   Group home _____

   Foster care _____

   Nursing home _____

   a. Available to people of normal intelligence who have developmental disabilities
   b. Must be licensed
   c. Congregate living
   d. Three to nine other residents
   e. No more than two other residents
   f. No limit on number of residents
   g. Could be ICF/MR

LESSON PLAN, SESSION 8: HABILITATION AND WORK

Competencies: I (H): Trainees will be able to discuss habilitation and work activities

    I (I): Trainees will know about support services

    I (J): Trainees will know where to find information about financial support

    I (K): Trainees will know about formal and informal support networks

Objectives: I (L): Trainees will be able to write a paragraph distinguishing between habilitation and work activities and discussing the importance of each

    I (M): Trainees will be able to list and describe modifications in programming for older clients of retirement age

    I (N): Given the words "advocacy," "guardianship," and "family support services" and a list of services, trainees will be able to match services to providers

    I (O): Trainees will be able to describe how a developmentally disabled person might be assisted to live in the community using only support services

Instructor	Trainee	Materials
Activity: Divide into small groups and do these activities	Participate in activity	Chalkboard or overhead projector and transparencies; if desired, copies of questions to be discussed
1. List as many well-known people as you can who have disabilities and what they do for a living		
2. List local people you know who have disabilities and who also earn a living and are relatively independent		
3. Combine the lists on chalkboard or transparency		
Discuss habilitation and work activities (Lecture Outline 8.I)	Take notes on lecture	Primary text, Chapter 9

(continued)

153

LESSON PLAN, SESSION 8: HABILITATION AND WORK (continued)

Instructor	Trainee	Materials
Activity: Return to small groups and discuss provisions for those individuals with developmental disabilities who are not yet independent or who require special services to become economically secure	Participate in activity	Chalkboard or overhead projector and transparencies; if desired, copies of questions to be discussed
1. Will some with normal intelligence always require sheltered or monitored employment?		
2. Is the sheltered workshop appropriate for those with DD who are not retarded?		
3. Are there advantages to the non-public agency sheltered workshops for those with DD?		
4. Combine answers on chalkboard or transparency		
Discuss support services (Lecture Outline 8.II)	Take notes on lecture	Primary text, Chapter 9
Distribute Activity Handout 1: "Case Studies"	List necessary and unnecessary support services for each case study	Activity Handout 1: "Case Studies"
Discuss financial support, formal and informal support networks (Lecture Outline 8.III, 8.IV)	Take notes on lecture	Primary text, Chapter 9

Evaluation: Have trainees write a paragraph distinguishing between habilitation and work activities

154

LECTURE OUTLINE 8: HABILITATION AND WORK

I. Work/habilitation services
    A. Employment
        1. Competitive employment puts the individual into the community in a job that is on the open market; for disabled workers, the work may be supervised by a staff person from an agency
        2. Sheltered employment is both work for pay (at a reduced rate based upon production) and for training, which occurs as part of the work experience
            a. Association for Persons with Severe Handicaps—goals for work/habilitation, pay, quality of working life, security benefits
            b. Same goals for disabled as for normal individuals
        3. Persons with DD other than retardation are eligible for sheltered employment in some workshops if they are certified "substantially developmentally disabled"
        4. Sheltered employment is also available through nonpublic agencies, such as UCP or Goodwill Industries in some areas
    B. Habilitation activities
        1. For a small number of DD individuals who are not able to work in sheltered employment, adult activity programs may meet the need for habilitation programming
        2. Part-time work: part-time classes are available in some settings to meet the needs of those who do not have the stamina to work whole days
        3. Special programs for retirement are needed
        4. ACCESS has designed a plan for community integration of older people with DD into community senior services
II. Support services
    A. Physical/health services
        1. Doctors, dentists, hospitals, clinics
        2. Services needed include: treatment of acute illness, medication supervision, surgery, long-term rehabilitation programs
        3. All medical personnel are not trained to work with people with developmental disabilities; look for those who can and will do it
    B. Specialized therapeutic interventions
        1. Occupational and physical therapists, speech therapists, psychologists
        2. Services include exercise, training, language remediation, behavior modification
        3. Persons with cerebral palsy have special needs for the services of OT, PT, and speech therapists
    C. Transportation/mobility
        1. Logistical support includes adaptive equipment for mobility: wheelchairs, braces, supports
        2. Aid in normalization of activities, getting to work, shopping, leisure activities
        3. Generic services should have adaptations for use with the handicapped, but few do; special transportation systems for the elderly and the handicapped exist in many communities

    D. Recreation and leisure
1. Some activities are provided by service agencies for their clients: parties, dances, trips
2. Community services are the most economical and normal to be accessed; Training and support may be needed; ACCESS is developing a system for facilitating such access to community services
3. Churches were found to be the only agencies reaching out to include the handicapped in the ACCESS study[1]

    E. Service coordination
1. If an individual with DD is served, an individualized habilitation plan (IHP) must be written and developed by an interdisciplinary team, including the DD individual and family
2. A case manager may be assigned to do individual program plan coordination for an agency

III. Financial support, Social Security, SSI: rules for eligibility are given in primary text; they may be discussed, if desired

IV. Formal support networks
    A. Advocacy
1. Case managers as advocates
2. Advocacy and protective services
3. Other nonpublic agencies are advocates for those who have the disability they focus on, for example, Epilepsy Foundation, Society for Autistic Citizens, United Cerebral Palsy

    B. Guardianship
1. Legal mechanism by which a disabled person can have decisions made and actions taken on his/her behalf
2. Guardianship information and advice may be secured from a lawyer

REFERENCE

1. Stroud, M., & Murphy, M. (1984). *The aged mentally retarded/developmentally disabled in Northeast Ohio.* ACCESS: Cooperative Planning for Service to Aged Mentally Retarded/Developmentally Disabled Persons. (Grant to The University of Akron from the Ohio Developmentally Disabled Planning Council, 84–25.)

CASE STUDIES

Consider the special needs of each person. List the kinds of support or services that would help each person lead a productive and satisfying life.

Sara

Sara is a 55-year-old woman with spina bifida who uses a wheelchair. She lives with her older brother and his wife in a large city. She would like to attend the local state university to learn how to use a computer so that she can get a part-time job doing billing for a medical group. Sara lives on a bus line, but the local buses have no lifts. She has SSI income of $345 per month. She wants to become more self-sufficient and would like to move to an apartment.

Donald

Donald is a 60-year-old who has epilepsy. He has light seizures three to four times a day. He attended school until fifth grade. He can read with great effort, but he makes a lot of mistakes and has difficulty understanding details of what he reads.

Since dropping out of school, he has had a number of service-type jobs: delivering packages (couldn't get them to the right places), filling hospital trays (got the wrong foods on them), and clerking in a grocery store (couldn't handle the money and give the right items for orders).

He is still living at home with his parents, largely because he has a lot of trouble managing his money and paying bills when they are due. He is in excellent health, very strong and good humored. He just isn't making it. His parents are in their 80s.

RESOURCE LIST

GENERAL INFORMATION

Janicki, M. P., & Jacobson, J. W. (1982). The character of developmental disabilities in New York state: Preliminary observations. *International Journal of Rehabilitation Research, 5*(2), 191–202.

Lubrin, R., Jacobson, J. W., & Keily, M. (1982). Projected impact of the functional definition of developmental disabilities: The categorically disabled population and service eligibility. *American Journal of Mental Deficiency, 87*(1), 73–79.

March of Dimes Birth Defects Foundation. *Public Health Education Information Sheets.* Available from author, 1275 Mamaronek Ave, White Plains, NY 10605.

AUTISM

Janicki, M. P., Lubrin, R. A., & Friedman, E. (1983). Variations in characteristics and service needs of persons with autism. *Journal of Autism and Developmental Disorders, 13*(1), 73–85.

Rabinovitch, R. D., & Pasley, F. C. *Early infantile autism: The clinical picture through adulthood* [Film]. Available from Film Office, Hawthorn Center, Northville, MI 48167, (313) 349-3000.

Autistic Children [Pamphlet]. Available from Institute of Child Behavior Research, Bernard Rimland, M.D., Director, 4157 Adams Ave., San Diego, CA 92116.

Volkman, F. R., & Cohen, D. J. (1982). A hierarchical analysis of patterns of non-compliance in autistic and behavior-disturbed children. *Journal of Autism and Developmental Disorders, 12*(1), 35–42.

EPILEPSY

Epilepsy [Film, 16mm]. Available from Abbott Laboratories Audio-Visual Services, 565 Fifth Ave., New York, NY 10017, (212) 986-0166.

How to recognize and classify seizures [Film]. Narrated by R. L. Masland, M.D. Available from Epilepsy Foundation of America, 1828 L Street, Washington, DC 20036. (Also available in videocassette.)

Epilepsy: Breaking down the walls of misunderstanding [Pamphlet]. Available from Public Affairs, Dept. 383 P, Abbott Laboratories, North Chicago, IL 60064. (Write to "Epilepsy Pamphlet"; enclose stamped, self-addressed envelope.)

DEVELOPMENTAL DISABILITIES

Epilepsy: Breaking down the walls of misunderstanding [Pamphlet]. Available from Public Affairs, Dept. 383 P, Abbott Laboratories, North Chicago, IL 60064. (Write to "Epilepsy Pamphlet"; enclose stamped, self-addressed envelope.)

How to recognize and classify seizures [Film]. Narrated by R. L. Masland, M.D. Available from Epilepsy Foundation of America, 1828 L Street, Washington, DC 20036. (Also available in videocassette.)

March of Dimes Birth Defects Foundation. *Public Health Information Sheets.* Available from author, 1275 Mamaronek Ave., White Plains, NY 10605.

Rabinovitch, R. D., & Pasley, F. C. *Early infantile autism: The clinical picture through adulthood.* Available from Film Office, Hawthorn Center, Northville, MI 48167, (313) 349-3000.

Autistic children. [Pamphlet]. Available from Institute for Child Behavior Research, Bernard Rimland, M.D., Director, 4157 Adams Ave., San Diego, CA 92116.

Planning for Community Access

COMPETENCIES

I. Knowledge: Trainees will know and be able to discuss accurately
    A. Legislative provisions or rules about retirement for older adults with developmental disabilities as illustrated by Ohio state policy
    B. Results of ACCESS research in terms of
        1. Percentages of older developmentally disabled adults in various kinds of programs
        2. Preferences of older developmentally disabled adults regarding use of time
    C. Options of developmentally disabled adults in use of time during later years
    D. Activity versus disengagement in later life
    E. Factors in successful aging; how older MR/DD adults compare with the general population in relation to these factors
    F. Concepts of group size in the accessing of community activities by older developmentally disabled adults
    G. Areas of social competence necessary to meet minimal community expectations
    H. Need for preassessment of clients chosen for access experience
    I. Content of ACCESS assessment tool
    J. Principles of planning for community access
    K. Variety of activities available within most communities
    L. How to assess appropriateness and suitability of activities with regard to safety, accessibility, social climate and expectations, program, and personnel
    M. Provisions of the Older Americans Act regarding senior programs
        1. Qualifications for participation in programs
        2. Types of programs provided
        3. Target populations
    N. Operation and characteristics of senior dining centers/nutrition sites
    O. Operation and characteristics of senior centers, adult day care centers, and senior social clubs
    P. Need for preplanning with agency personnel
    Q. Importance of acceptance of MR/DD adults by nonhandicapped members of programs or groups
    R. How negative feelings are acquired toward minority populations with whom one does not regularly associate
    S. How feelings deter the process of planning and innovative programming for the minority population
    T. Common feelings of MR/DD adults accessing new situations

    U.   Ways in which personnel of community-based activities can contribute toward successful access of those activities by older MR/DD adults

    V.   How the consortium process can benefit planning and access

II. Skills: Trainees will be able to

    A.   Identify community-based programs specifically planned for older persons

    B.   Identify other community-based programs and activity options that are age and level appropriate for older MR/DD adults

    C.   Identify community-based activities that would provide interesting and appropriate experiences for older MR/DD adults

    D.   Assess individual client readiness for accessing community-based activities

    E.   Select activities based on assessment for training/preparation for the community accessing experience

    F.   Identify steps in planning for access to community-based activities

    G.   Assess appropriateness of a community-based activity

        1. Site safety and assessibility

        2. Program

        3. Expectations

        4. Staff

    H.   Plan with an agency or group director for a community accessing experience for an older MR/DD adult

    I.   Understand feelings of personnel of community-based activities who are asked to accept older MR/DD clients

    J.   Assist those personnel to work successfully with older MR/DD adults

    K.   Participate in a group planning process that brings together representatives of different service systems with mutual concerns

OBJECTIVES

I. Knowledge: Trainees will

    A.   List legislative provisions in own state pertaining to retirement and special programs for older persons with developmental disabilities

    B.   List three preferences for use of leisure time described in *The Aged Mentally Retarded/Developmentally Disabled in Northeast Ohio*[1]

    C.   List 10–12 *possible* options for leisure/recreation activities for an older person with developmental disabilities

    D.   Given a list of factors that appear to lead to successful aging, identify those that apply to older persons with mental retardation/developmental disability

    E.   Given a hypothetical situation involving large group access to a community event, list two positive and three negative aspects or possible outcomes

    F.   Given a hypothetical situation involving small group or individual access to a community event, list four positive potential outcomes

    G.   List three areas of social competence necessary to meet community expectations

    H.   List eight principles of planning for community access

    I.   Given a description of a specific community activity site, assess same in terms of safety, accessibility, social climate, rules, expectations, appropriateness of program, personnel

    J.   List four major services that have been established under the Older Americans Act

    K.   Write a paragraph comparing nutrition sites, senior centers, adult day care centers, and senior social clubs to each other in terms of organization, funding, leadership, and function

    L.   Prepare an agenda for a meeting of a leader of developmentally disabled adult services and a senior club director to plan an accessing experience for an older developmentally disabled person

    M.   Write a paragraph describing how feelings may deter the process of successful planning for access and the accessing process itself

    N.   List three ways in which personnel of community-based activities can facilitate successful access of an older developmentally disabled person

II.   Skills: Trainees will be able to

    A.   Assess readiness of a client for community activity using ACCESS assessment form (Appendix 10.A, primary text)

    B.   Identify clients' needs for specialized training based on assessment

    C.   Given a list of interests of an older developmentally disabled person, design a set of 10 appropriate community-based activities for that person

    D.   Assess appropriateness of one community-based activity, using checklist (Figure 11.1, p. 110, primary text)

    E.   Suggest and demonstrate ways to alleviate or overcome negative feelings toward persons with developmental disabilities

REFERENCE

1.   Stroud, M., & Murphy, M. (1984). *The aged mentally retarded/developmentally disabled in Northeast Ohio*. ACCESS: Cooperative Planning for Service to Aged Mentally Retarded/Developmentally Disabled Persons. (Grant to The University of Akron from the Ohio Developmental Disabilities Planning Council, 84-25.)

LESSON PLAN, SESSION 1: WHY RETIREMENT? WHY ACCESS?

Competencies: I (A): Trainees will know and be able to discuss legislative provisions or rules about retirement for older adults with DD as illustrated by Ohio state policy

I (B): Trainees will know and be able to discuss results of ACCESS research with regard to percentages of older adults with DD in various programs and preferences of these adults regarding use of time

I (C): Trainees will know and be able to discuss options of adults with DD in use of time during later years

I (D): Trainees will know and be able to discuss activity versus disengagement in later life

I (E): Trainees will know and be able to discuss factors in successful aging, and how adults with MR/DD compare with the general population in relation to these factors

II (A): Trainees will be able to identify community-based programs specifically planned for older persons

II (B): Trainees will be able to identify other community-based programs and activity options that are age and level appropriate for older MR/DD adults

II (C): Trainees will be able to identify community-based activities that would provide interesting and appropriate experiences for older MR/DD adults

Objectives: I (A): Trainees will list legislative provisions in own state pertaining to retirement and special programs for older persons with DD

I (B): Trainees will list three preferences for use of leisure time described in *The Aged Mentally Retarded/Developmentally Disabled in Northeast Ohio*

I (C): Trainees will list 10–12 *possible* options for leisure/recreation activities for an older person with DD

I (D): Given a list of factors that appear to lead to successful aging, trainees will identify those that apply to older persons with MR/DD

Instructor	Trainee	Materials
Discuss retirement in normal and MR/DD persons (Lecture Outline 1.I, 1.II)	Take notes on lecture	Primary text, Overview (Section III)
Ask the trainee to describe any Older Americans programs that they know of which include older MR/DD persons	Describe existing programs, personal experiences	
Discuss theories of aging (Lecture Outline 1.III)		
Introduce film: *Aging*	View film	Film: *Aging*; projector
Lead discussion about film: life-styles in retirement	Discuss	
Introduce videotape/filmstrip: *Hey Look at Me*	View filmstrip	Videotape/filmstrip: *Hey Look At Me*; tape or strip player
Lead discussion following filmstrip: life-styles of older adults with developmental disabilities	Discuss three life-styles shown: How do they differ? How are they alike? Which would be easiest to include in senior activities? Which would require more training? How do they compare with "normal" population?	
Organize class into dyads and discuss "What I'd like to do when I reach retirement age"	Participate in dyad discussions	

Evaluation: Have class develop at least three alternative retirement options for older adults with DD in outline form

163

LECTURE OUTLINE 1: THEORIES AND PHILOSOPHIES OF AGING/RETIREMENT

I. Retirement in normal life span
   A. Men and women now have the opportunity to work until age 70
   B. Many still choose to retire from work at age 55, 60, 65; others are interested in working as long as possible
   C. Many companies promote early retirement; others would prefer to retain their experienced workers
   D. Two trends are observed in the "retirement years":
      1. Those who take a good pension and early retirement and concentrate on enjoying family and leisure activities
      2. Those who prefer to continue working in a full- or part-time capacity, sometimes beginning a new career
   E. Typically retirement brings changes in life-style, finances, role identity, amount of leisure, structuring of time, and sometimes health
II. Retirement and the older MR/DD person
   A. Retirement has only recently become an option for older adults in some states, for example:
      1. New rules of the Ohio Department of MR/DD instruct the County Boards as follows:

> Although no mandatory retirement is required, adults 55 and over who no longer desire a program emphasizing work skills training and employment shall have available to them a retirement program emphasizing leisure time, nutrition and health, exercise, community integration, and other training components. (Ohio Revised Code 5123:2-2-06)

   B. Research[1] indicates that many older MR/DD persons are still employed in sheltered work
   C. Preferences indicated by older persons in this research are: part-time work, social activities, new programs
   D. In northeast Ohio a few county boards have organized programs for older clients and designated special staff who develop alternative programming[2]
   E. Choices in activities during their later years are the right of the older MR/DD person
      1. New experiences, personal growth, and learning may be among those choices
      2. Activities preparatory to access or inclusion in community-based activities may be part of later life activities
III. Theories of aging
   A. Disengagement theory based on the Kansas City studies of the late 1950s proposes that everyone is innately programmed for withdrawal from the mainstream in the later years of life (65 +)
   B. Later theories challenged this idea and proposed that activity in later life is most appropriate and essential to maintenance of function
   C. More recent theories indicate many different aging styles and preferred life-styles, including disengagement and various levels of activity

D. Gerontological studies indicate these possible factors in successful aging:
   1. Good health
   2. Financial security
   3. Feeling of usefulness
   4. Strong social network

REFERENCES

1. Stroud, M., & Murphy, M. (1984). *The aged mentally retarded/developmentally disabled in Northeast Ohio*. ACCESS: Cooperative Planning for Service to Aged Mentally Retarded/Developmentally Disabled Persons. (Grant to The University of Akron from the Ohio Developmental Disabilities Planning Council, No. 84-25.)
2. Herrera, P. (1983). *Innovative programming for the aging & aged mentally retarded/developmentally disabled adult*. Akron, OH: Exploration Press.

LESSON PLAN, SESSION 2: PREPARING FOR COMMUNITY ACCESS

Competencies: I (F): Trainees will know and be able to discuss concepts of group size in the accessing of community activities by older DD adults

    I (G): Trainees will know and be able to discuss areas of social competence necessary to meet minimal community expectations

    I (H): Trainees will know and be able to discuss the need for preassessment of clients chosen for access experience
    I (I): Trainees will know and be able to discuss the content of the ACCESS assessment tool
    II (D): Trainees will be able to assess individual client readiness for accessing community-based activities
    II (E): Trainees will be able to select activities based on assessment, for training/preparation for the community accessing experience

Objectives: I (E): Trainees will be able to identify steps in planning for access to community-based activities
    I (E): Given a hypothetical situation involving large group access to a community event, trainees will list two positive and three negative aspects or possible outcomes
    I (F): Given a hypothetical situation involving small group or individual access to a community event, trainees will list four positive potential outcomes
    I (G): Trainees will list three areas of social competence necessary to meet community expectations
    I (H): Trainees will list eight principles of planning for community access
    II (A): Trainees will be able to assess readiness of a client for community activity using ACCESS assessment form
    II (B): Trainees will be able to identify client's needs for specialized training based on assessment results
    II (C): Given a list of interest of an older DD person, trainees will be able to design a set of 10 appropriate community-based activities for that person

Instructor	Trainee	Materials
Discuss concepts of group size in the access of community activities by MR/DD adults	Listen and take notes	Primary text, Chapter 10
Divide students into small groups; let each group decide what the	Participate in group discussion	Prompting questions on 3 × 5 cards

Content	Action	Resources
community expectations (limits) are for an older and/or MR/DD person in each of these areas 1. Behavior toward others 2. Appearance 3. Observing rules and regulations 4. Conversational skills		
Lead summarizing reports	Group member gives report	Chalkboard or flipchart
Present facts about discrimination, need for meeting community expectations (Lecture Outline 2A)	Take notes on lecture	Primary text, Chapter 10
Present ACCESS assessment form, discuss its use in preassessment of clients; ask students to practice assessment of an older MR/DD person, then to design 1. Individualized program to improve deficits in preparation for access 2. A community-based activity program based on person's interests (10 activities)	If possible, complete an assessment of an older adult with MR/DD outside of class and design programs	Handout 1: "ACCESS Assessment of Older Adults with Developmental Disabilities"
Discuss principles of planning for community access	Listen and take notes	Primary text, Chapter 10
Organize debate about using volunteers	Present pro and con issues about the use of volunteers with MR/DD adults	Brochures from various volunteer agencies
Present basics of volunteer administration (Lecture Outline 2B)	Listen and take notes	Primary text, Chapter 10

Evaluation: Have group make a checklist for leaders preparing to take clients to a community activity; list should include community site contacts, expectations, relevant information from ACCESS Assessment

LECTURE OUTLINE 2A: DISCRIMINATION AND COMMUNITY EXPECTATIONS

  I.   Communities set standards for acceptable and unacceptable behavior and appearance
       A.   Community size may affect these unwritten limitations
       B.   Geographic location may affect them
       C.   Limitations/expectations may reflect other aspects of the social milieu
 II.   Our society is more tolerant of youth in general in enforcing these limitations than it is of certain minority groups: the aged, developmentally disabled, races other than Caucasian
III.   Developmentally disabled older persons must be helped to achieve social expectations if they are to participate in community-based activities

ACCESS Assessment of Older Adults with Developmental Disabilities

(Confidential)

Name _____ **DOB** _____ **M** ____ **F** ____ **ID** _____

Program
    Enrollment _____

    Site address _____ Phone _____

    Contact person _____ Phone _____

Residence
    Own family ____ Group home ____ Indep ____ Nursing home ____ Devel. ctr. ____

    Address _____

    Contact person _____ Phone _____

    Relationship or position _____

    Number in household ____ Sources of income _____

    Monthly income _____

MR level _____ **Adaptive behavior level** _____ **Religious preference** _____

Guardian _____ **Type** _____

Data collector _____ **Agency** _____

    Position _____ Phone _____

Data sources
    Individual interview _____   Individual habilitation plan _____

    Caregiver interview _____   Staff of residential facility _____

    Case manager _____   Family, relative _____

PHYSICAL CONDITION

	Average	Weak	Impaired	Disabled	Comment
General health	4	3	2	1	_____
Vision	4	3	2	1	_____
Hearing	4	3	2	1	_____
Teeth	4	3	2	1	_____
Limbs	4	3	2	1	_____
Joints	4	3	2	1	_____

	Doesn't need	Uses	Has, doesn't use	Needs	
Eyeglasses	4	3	2	1	_____
Hearing aid	4	3	2	1	_____
Dentures	4	3	2	1	_____
Cane/walker	4	3	2	1	_____
Wheelchair	4	3	2	1	_____

ACCESS Assessment

Chronic conditions	Medication	Schedule
___ Heart disease	_____	_____
___ Circulatory	_____	_____
___ Seizures	_____	_____
___ Diabetes	_____	_____
___ Parkinson	_____	_____
___ Cerebral palsy	_____	_____
___ Cancer	_____	_____
___ Ulcer	_____	_____
___ Other: _____	_____	_____
_____	_____	_____

Nutrition

Status, weight   Underweight _____ Normal _____ Overweight _____ Obese _____

Special diet _____

Food texture _____

SOCIAL COMPETENCIES

Self-Care and ADL	Independent	Verbal cue	Assistance	Unable	Comments
Walking	4	3	2	1	_____
Grooming	4	3	2	1	_____
Eating	4	3	2	1	_____
Climbing stairs	4	3	2	1	_____
Toileting	4	3	2	1	_____
Transferring	4	3	2	1	_____
Dressing	4	3	2	1	_____
Using telephone	4	3	2	1	_____
Using public transportation	4	3	2	1	_____
Finding way around community	4	3	2	1	_____
Make purchases	4	3	2	1	_____
Housekeeping	4	3	2	1	_____
Doing laundry	4	3	2	1	_____
Taking own medication	4	3	2	1	_____
Bathing/handwashing	4	3	2	1	_____

Social interactions	About right	Passive	Too much	Withdrawn	
With staff	4	3	2	1	_____
With peers	4	3	2	1	_____
With family, relatives	4	3	2	1	_____
With professionals	4	3	2	1	_____
With strangers	4	3	2	1	_____

Relationships	Many	Some	Few	None	
Friends among staff	4	3	2	1	_____
Among peers at work, home	4	3	2	1	_____
Relatives seen frequently	4	3	2	1	_____

ACCESS Assessment

People in community/ advocate	4	3	2	1	_____
Affectionate relation- ship	4	3	2	1	_____

Maladaptive behaviors	Rare, never	Sometimes	Frequent	Problematic	
Verbal aggression	4	3	2	1	_____
Physical aggression	4	3	2	1	_____
Refusal to participate	4	3	2	1	_____
Socially inappropri- ate	4	3	2	1	_____
Self-injurious	4	3	2	1	_____
Withdrawn	4	3	2	1	_____
Stealing	4	3	2	1	_____
Property destruction	4	3	2	1	_____
Fearful, anxious	4	3	2	1	_____
Depressed	4	3	2	1	_____
Disoriented	4	3	2	1	_____
Wanders away	4	3	2	1	_____

Behavior programs _____

COGNITIVE FUNCTIONING

Communication	Normal or nearly	Phrases	Single words	Gesture	Comments
Expressive language	4	3	2	1	_____
Receptive language	4	3	2	1	_____
Intelligibility	4	3	2	1	_____

Functional Academics	Independent	Some help	Much help	None	
Reads menu, pro- gram sentences	4	3	2	1	_____
Reads "survival words"	4	3	2	1	_____
Writes words, sentences	4	3	2	1	_____
Tells time	4	3	2	1	_____
Uses currency, coins	4	3	2	1	_____
Makes change	4	3	2	1	_____
Uses calendar	4	3	2	1	_____

LEISURE AND RECREATION ACTIVITIES INTERVIEW

4—Often   3—Sometimes
2—Rarely   1—Never

Leisure (at home)	Comments	Would you like to?
Television		4 3 2 1
Table games		4 3 2 1
Active games		4 3 2 1
Exercises		4 3 2 1
Gardening, house plants		4 3 2 1

(continued)

ACCESS Assessment

Household chores	4 3 2 1
Taking walks, hikes	4 3 2 1
Knit/crochet/needlework	4 3 2 1
Woodwork, craft	4 3 2 1
Collecting	4 3 2 1
Drawing or painting	4 3 2 1
Listening to music	4 3 2 1
Outdoor sports	4 3 2 1
Looking at books/magazines	4 3 2 1
Photography	4 3 2 1
Keeping a pet	4 3 2 1
Chatting with friends	4 3 2 1
Cooking	4 3 2 1

Recreation (in community)

Going out to eat	4 3 2 1
Bowling	4 3 2 1
Movies, shows	4 3 2 1
Sporting events	4 3 2 1
Shopping	4 3 2 1
Museums, exhibits	4 3 2 1
Church, worship/social event	4 3 2 1
Musical show or concert	4 3 2 1
Dancing, parties	4 3 2 1
Special interest group	4 3 2 1
Swimming	4 3 2 1
Camping	4 3 2 1
Live shows	4 3 2 1
Senior center	4 3 2 1
Travelogues	4 3 2 1
Fairs, carnivals	4 3 2 1
Amusement parks	4 3 2 1
Lectures, speakers	4 3 2 1
Going to visit someone	4 3 2 1
Walking around a mall	4 3 2 1
Classes	4 3 2 1
Fishing	4 3 2 1
Parks	4 3 2 1
Other	4 3 2 1

ACCESS Assessment

COMMUNITY SERVICES AND PROVIDERS

Co. Bd. of MR/DD _____

Residential services _____

Mental health services _____

Rehabilitation services _____

Advocacy/guardianship _____

Transportation _____

Church _____

Legal services/attorney _____

Senior Center/nutrition site _____

Home-delivered meals _____

Homemaker services _____

Adult day care _____

Senior Friends _____

Medical services _____

Physician _____

Dentist _____

Medical equipment _____

Speech therapy _____

Occupational therapy _____

Physical therapy _____

Podiatrist _____

Pharmacy _____

Other _____

ADDITIONAL COMMENTS

_____

_____

_____

_____

_____

_____

_____

_____

Information from assessment given to:

Agency   **Date**

_____   _____

_____   _____

_____   _____

_____   _____

(*continued*)

ACCESS Assessment

Recommendations

_____

_____

_____

_____

_____

Participation in ACCESS Program

_____

_____

_____

(ACCESS Assessment Form developed through **ACCESS: Cooperative Planning for Services to Aged Persons with Developmental Disabilities,** Ohio Development Disabilities Planning Council Grant 84-25, and **Community Access for Elderly Mentally Retarded Persons,** a grant from the Joseph P. Kennedy, Jr. Foundation. Ruth Roberts, Ph.D., Director, Marion Stroud, Ph.D., Research Director, Evelyn Sutton, M.A., Gerontologist, and Gary A. Davis, B.A., Field Coordinator, The University of Akron.)

LECTURE OUTLINE 2B: VOLUNTEER ADMINISTRATION

I. The use of volunteers is highly recommended as a means of expanding quality and quantity of service to clients in residences, workshops, or other programs for the developmentally disabled

II. Value of volunteer service is proportional to the amount of time invested in management of a volunteer program

III. Volunteer management includes five basic areas
    A. Recruitment
        1. Job descriptions
        2. Circulation of need for volunteers through appropriate channels
        3. Application process, usually including information form, referrals
    B. Interviews/screening
        1. In-depth one-to-one
        2. Exploration of motives, expectations, limitations of the volunteer
        3. Exploration of special interests, skills, experience of the volunteer
        4. In-depth description of agency, clients, volunteer responsibilities, supervisory process
        5. Decision regarding suitability of volunteer applicant for position
        6. Arrangement of next steps
    C. Training to include
        1. Physical plant of the agency (tour)
        2. Introduction to appropriate personnel
        3. Policies of the agency
        4. Attitude training (toward clients, professionals)
        5. Details of the volunteer job
        6. Special skills and techniques required (in-depth)
        7. Other appropriate information
    D. Placement
        1. Introduction of the volunteer to the job
        2. On-the-job supervision and training
    E. Evaluation—interview at appropriate intervals to determine success of placement, ongoing needs for training
    F. Recognition
        1. Formal
        2. Informal

LESSON PLAN, SESSION 3: APPROPRIATE COMMUNITY-BASED ACTIVITIES

Competencies: I (K): Trainees will know and be able to discuss the variety of activities available within most communities

I (L): Trainees will know and be able to discuss how to assess appropriateness and suitability of activities

I (M): Trainees will know and be able to discuss the provisions of the Older Americans Act

I (N): Trainees will know and be able to discuss the operation and characteristics of senior dining centers/nutrition sites

I (O): Trainees will know and be able to discuss the operation and characteristics of senior centers, adult day care centers, and senior social clubs

I (P): Trainees will know and be able to discuss the need for preplanning with agency personnel

II (G): Trainees will be able to assess appropriateness of a community-based activity

II (H): Trainees will be able to plan with an agency or group director for a community access experience for an older MR/DD adult

Objectives: I (I): Given a description of a specific community activity site, trainees will assess same

I (J): Trainees will list four major services that have been established under the Older Americans Act

I (K): Trainees will write a paragraph comparing nutrition sites, senior centers, adult day care centers, and senior social clubs to each other

I (L): Trainees will prepare an agenda for a meeting of a leader of DD adult services and a senior club director to plan an accessing experience for an older DD person

II (D): Trainees will be able to assess appropriateness of a community-based activity, using checklist in primary text

Instructor	Trainee	Materials
Introduce concept of community-based activities (Lecture Outline 3A)		Primary text, Chapter 11
Present list of activities for older people in community, ask for additions	Add ideas to expand activities list	Copies of Exhibit 11.1 (primary text, p. 110)

176

Present concept of assessing appropri-ateness of community-based activities; introduce checklist	Individually assess a possible site	Copies of Figure 11.1 (primary text, p. 111)
Identify activities and services provided by Older Americans Act		
Introduce subject of nutrition sites; have students read about nutrition sites; ask for critical comment from anyone present who has first-hand experience	Independent study	Primary text, Chapter 11; flyers, brochures from various local nutrition sites
Present information about senior centers (if class includes senior center directors, ask them to describe their settings and programs), adult day care centers, and senior social clubs	Listen and take notes	Primary text, Chapter 11
Summarize principles of planning for community access; ask students to develop agenda for cooperative planning meeting (Lecture Outline 3B)	Design agenda	Primary text, Chapter 11; chalkboard

Evaluation: Have trainees locate and list addresses and phone numbers for at least one local site for each of the following senior activities: nutrition site, senior center, adult day care, senior social club

LECTURE OUTLINE 3A: COMMUNITY-BASED ACTIVITIES

I. In the context of this training, community-based activities and services are those sponsored by agencies, churches, and nonprofit or for-profit organizations in community settings that are open to all, or that have qualifications for participation that can be met by an older MR/DD person
   A. Generic (available to the general public, nonprofit)
       1. Churches, church groups, and events
       2. Parks, recreation areas, beaches
       3. Nature and environmental centers
       4. Observatories
       5. Camp grounds, lakes, fishing spots
       6. Hobby groups
       7. Continuing education centers
       8. Libraries, museums, galleries
       9. Craft shows, art shows
       10. Ethnic fairs, community celebrations, county fairs, dog shows
       11. High-school plays, community theater
       12. Greenhouses, gardens, historic homes
       13. Horse farm, zoo
       14. Campus
       15. Industry, newspaper, phone company
   B. Generic (for profit)
       1. Swimming pool
       2. Bowling alley
       3. Amusement park
       4. Movie
       5. Restaurant
       6. Game center
       7. Night club
       8. Shopping mall
       9. Concerts, dramatic productions
       10. Sporting events: ball games, tennis matches, etc.
       11. Sightseeing tours
   C. Specifically senior
       1. Dining centers (nutrition sites)
       2. Senior centers
       3. Senior club
       4. Senior programs sponsored by city or county recreation department

LECTURE OUTLINE 3B: PLANNING FOR SUCCESSFUL ACCESS: SUMMARY

I. Motivation for providing opportunities for older MR/DD people to access community-based activities
   A. To help them experience new and different environments
   B. To assist them in expanding their social networks and support systems
   C. To increase their range of leisure time options
   D. To facilitate their utilization of existing programs for older adults
   E. To help them achieve personal growth in later years of life

II. Important considerations for those who facilitate community access for older MR/DD persons
   A. Few is better
   B. Community expectations
   C. Appropriateness of selected activities
   D. Careful appraisal of setting(s) to be accessed
   E. Personal contact with community personnel
   F. Identification of strengths and weaknesses of individual MR/DD older person
   G. Provision for decision-making opportunities
   H. Use of volunteer assistants
      1. In preparatory activities (e.g., conversational skills practice)
      2. As peer companions, escorts

LESSON PLAN, SESSION 4: UNDERSTANDING AND MEETING COMMUNITY EXPECTATIONS AND BARRIERS

Competencies: I (Q): Trainees will know and be able to discuss importance of acceptance of MR/DD adults by nonhandicapped members of programs or groups

I (R): Trainees will know and be able to discuss how negative feelings are acquired toward minority populations with whom one does not regularly associate

I (S): Trainees will know and be able to discuss how feelings deter the process of planning and innovative programming for the minority population

I (T): Trainees will know and be able to discuss common feelings of MR/DD adults accessing new situations

I (U): Trainees will know and be able to discuss ways in which personnel of community-based activities can contribute toward successful access of those activities by older MR/DD adults

II (I): Trainees will be able to understand feelings of personnel of community-based activities who are asked to accept older MR/DD clients

II (J): Trainees will be able to assist those personnel to work successfully with older MR/DD adults

Objectives: I (M): Trainees will write a paragraph describing how feelings may deter the process of successful planning for access and the accessing process itself

II (E): Trainees will be able to suggest and demonstrate ways to alleviate or overcome negative feelings toward persons with DD

Instructor	Trainee	Materials
Organize students into small groups; distribute Activity Handout 1A: "The Community Center Board Meeting"; Activity Handout 1B: "A Party at the Nursing Home"; Activity Handout 1C: "Look Who Wants to Move In!" (each group to have one handout)	Participate in simulations	Primary text, Chapter 11; Activity Handout 1A: "The Community Center Board Meeting"; Activity Handout 1B: "A Party at the Nursing Home"; Activity Handout 1C: "Look Who Wants to Move In!"
Record major points of reports on blackboard	Report on results of simulations	Blackboard
Organize students into small groups; distribute Activity Handout 2: "Role Play"	Follow Activity Handout 2 instructions; participate in role play	Activity Handout 2: "Role Play" descriptions of situations on 3 × 5 cards
Lead summary discussion on *feelings* and *attitudes* of clients, staff of agencies, public that may affect access planning	Participate in discussion	
Lead discussion of suggestions found in primary text, Chapter 12, p. 120	Discuss, delete, and/or add ideas	Primary text, Chapter 12

Evaluation: Evaluate the simulations as a total group; identify obstructions as well as good solutions; discuss methods of dealing with negative opinions

THE COMMUNITY CENTER BOARD MEETING

You are an older adult who is on the Board of Advisors to the local Senior Citizens' Center. Your Center has a well-rounded program for seniors, including a nutrition program, exercises, table games, field trips, concerts, a Seniors Band, and evening programs like lectures or travel films. You also have an active group who do all sorts of charitable work in the community.

The Director of Adult Services at the County Board of Mental Retardation program has written a request to the Board to include the older MR/DD adults in the Senior Center Program. You need to discuss the proposal and come to some decisions about this request.

Do you want to include them?
How many can you handle?
How can you talk to those people?
Do they really belong there?
Will others stay home if the MR/DD kind come?
Should you expect dangerous behavior?
Do they make your "normal" people nervous?
What kinds of activities might they do?
Will they act funny?
Won't they be better off with their own kind?
Can they eat in public?

These and many other concerns occur to the members of the Board. Please choose a reporter to bring your conclusions back to the whole group.

NOTES

_____
_____
_____
_____
_____
_____
_____
_____
_____

"Experts" on both aging and mental retardation will be available for consultation with your group—but only your group can make decisions.

A PARTY AT THE NURSING HOME

You are a senior citizen who lives in a large multiunit nursing home. You and a number of other residents are planning a Halloween party for the nursing home. One unit of the home is occupied by mentally retarded persons who were formerly residents of an institution. All are over 60. They are usually left out of the activities for "normal" persons, but this time their activities staff have requested that they be included in the party. You need to decide whether to honor that request, and if so, what terms you will set and what preparations you will make. Please choose someone to be the head nurse of the MR/DD unit, and someone to be head nurse of the ordinary older people. They will need to make reports.

Would they upset the others?
It is possible to talk to them?
Could they participate in activities?
Could they help in the planning?
How could each group be prepared for the other group?
Is that necessary?
Can they behave like normal people?
Are you afraid of some of their possible behaviors?
Can they wear costumes?
Could they sing?

The "normals" nurse should be opposed.

NOTES

_____

_____

_____

_____

_____

_____

_____

_____

_____

_____

_____

"Experts" from the fields of MR/DD and aging are available to you for consultation.

LOOK WHO WANTS TO MOVE IN!

You are a senior citizen who is a member of the Housing Admissions Committee at the place where you live, a multiunit apartment building complex. You are reviewing an application from an older mentally retarded couple. They are married to each other, so you don't have a morals problem, but you have some concerns. . . .

Can people like that get married?
How do they manage their money?
How do they get money?
Who shops for them?
Do they have friends like themselves?
Can they be trusted?
What if they leave their gas on and cause a fire?
Will they embarrass the others?
Will others want to move out?
Do they carry AIDS or some other diseases?

These and other concerns can be discussed. You might want to think of the kinds of things you'd have to do to prepare them or other tenants for the move. Appoint a chairperson to report to the whole group.

NOTES

_____
_____
_____
_____
_____
_____
_____
_____
_____
_____
_____

"Experts" in both MR/DD and aging are available to consult with your group, but only the group can make any decisions.

ROLE PLAY

Divide into small groups to prepare and present two or more of the following:

1. Retarded older person on first visit to senior center gets warm, reinforcing welcome.
2. Retarded older person on first visit to senior center gets (much) less than warm, reinforcing welcome.
3. Inexperienced senior club director exhibits nervousness and lack of confidence in dealing with newcomer who is developmentally disabled.
4. Senior club director exhibits knowledge and understanding in dealing with newcomer who is developmentally disabled.
5. Two or three staff members of senior nutrition sites mask and/or express their real feelings in discussing plans for access of two developmentally disabled older adults with their group home leader.

LESSON PLAN, SESSION 5: BRINGING SERVICE SYSTEMS TOGETHER

Competency: I (V): Trainees will know and be able to discuss how the consortium process can benefit planning and access
Objective: I (N): Trainees will list three ways in which personnel of community-based activities can facilitate successful access of an older adult with developmental disabilities

Instructor	Trainee	Materials
Present information or (preferred) introduce guest presenters to describe funding, structure, jurisdiction, etc. of MR/DD and aging (federal, state, local) service systems	Listen and take notes	Primary text, Appendix B
Ask trainees to diagram structure of each system; compile diagrams into single diagram for each system	Draw diagrams of aging and MR/DD service systems; present	Chalkboard or flipchart
Lead discussion comparing structure and funding of the two systems	Participate in discussion	
Ask: "What communication problems might representatives of the two systems have when meeting together?"	Respond	

Request examples of terminology, language, jargon, acronyms, etc. that might prove a barrier to communication; list on chalkboard in two columns	Give examples	Chalkboard or flipchart
Organize small groups to discuss: "What issues/problems might the two systems have in common?"	Participate in small groups	
Conduct feedback session; add to list as needed	Give feedback	
Ask trainees to suggest agencies from each system who might profitably join together to plan for services for older MR/DD clients; list on chalkboard	Suggest agencies	Chalkboard or flipchart
Present information on the Consortium model (Lecture Outline 5), and summarize		Primary text, Appendix B

Evaluation: List as individuals or group three ways in which personnel of community-based activities can facilitate access of older adults with DD

LECTURE OUTLINE 6: THE CONSORTIUM: A PLANNING MODEL

I.   The Consortium, a cooperative planning model applied to MR/DD and aging
    A.   Definition of consortium
    B.   Appropriate agencies to be included
    C.   Organizational steps involved
        1.   Role of leadership
        2.   Assessment of need/interest
        3.   Initial invitation and mailing list
        4.   Initial agenda
            a.   Getting acquainted
            b.   Presentations
            c.   Research questions; future directions
            d.   Consensus regarding next steps

II. Values/benefits of Consortium model in planning services for older MR/DD clients
    A.   Efficiency in saving time, resources, duplication, etc.
    B.   Improvement in quality of service to clients
    C.   Possible new services and programs
    D.   Possible training
    E.   Possible new projects
    F.   Advocacy development
    G.   Information sharing
    H.   Benefits of networking; new colleagues
    I.   Pursuing areas of joint interest (e.g., nutrition, housing, geriatric assessment, elder abuse)
    J.   Personal (individual) growth

AUDIOVISUAL RESOURCES

Aging (21 min.), color, 1973, H,C,A,S; (Educational Psychology Series): Examines some popular, yet commonly mistaken, attitudes toward the aged and their place in society. Discusses two major theories on the aged—the Activity Theory and the Disengagement Theory—and the research being done by Bernice Neugarten, Robert Havighurst, and Sheldon Tobin, of the University of Chicago. Discussion guide.

Hey Look At Me (15 min.), color videotape , 1980: University of Michigan; produced in cooperation with Macomb/Oakland Regional Center and Michigan Department of Mental Health.

Discipline with Dignity

How to Work with Dependent Adults

COMPETENCIES

I. Knowledge: Trainees will know and be able to discuss accurately
    A. What maladaptive behaviors are, giving examples, and how they are counterproductive
    B. Some physiological, social, and personal explanations for maladaptive behaviors in older dependent adults
    C. Some environmental changes that can be made to prevent occurrences of maladaptive behaviors
    D. Recommended training methods for teaching socially acceptable behaviors and practicing them
    E. Why punishment is counterproductive and discipline involving decision making based upon choice is preferable
    F. The use of least intrusive intervention techniques to prevent escalation of behavior problems
    G. Conversational techniques that encourage cooperation and preserve the dignity of others
    H. The names and some features of specialized strategies for dealing with individuals and small groups
II. Skills: Trainees will be able to
    A. Identify maladaptive behaviors
    B. Make a checklist to evaluate an environment
    C. Design a plan with objectives and activities for a group meeting of dependent adults
    D. Develop a model for instruction in socially acceptable behavior using either live modeling, videotaping, audiotaping, or photos
    E. Demonstrate intervention strategies that prevent escalation of maladaptive behaviors
    F. Use the conversational strategies that preserve dignity
III. Attitude: Trainees will
    A. Consciously treat others in ways that preserve their dignity
    B. Use methods of working with others that provide maximum self-control and avoid punishment or embarrassment
    C. Where possible, correct the environmental causes or help the individual with physiological or social problems to improve rather than merely deal with behaviors

D. Talk to dependent adults and others respectfully, using the techniques given in the module whenever possible

OBJECTIVES

I. Knowledge: Trainees will
   A. After discussion, list at least eight maladaptive behaviors and tell how they are annoying, counterproductive, or harmful to others
   B. After instruction, list possible causes of maladaptive behavior in these categories: physiological, learned, psychological (frustration, loss, mental illness), and social (frustration, low self-esteem, deprivations of basic needs)
   C. Describe an instructional program for a group of older adults that uses either modeling or small group work to teach a socially acceptable behavior
   D. Give at least five reasons that punishment is counterproductive as a way of controlling behavior in others
   E. Identify the elements needed for self-discipline as discussed by Dreikurs: freedom to choose how to act, understanding what results of actions are likely to be, and ability to make decisions
   F. Given a situation where maladaptive behaviors are portrayed in a sociodrama or a videotaped episode, suggest three intervention strategies proposed by Redl and modified for this module
   G. In a role play, respond to statements or requests in ways that preserve dignity and show respect
II. Skills: Trainees will be able to
   A. In either a simulated situation or viewing a videotape, identify maladaptive behaviors when they are displayed
   B. Identify elements in a given environment that might lead to maladaptive behaviors and recommend modifications
   C. Given the need to train clients in a specific behavior, prepare lesson plans with objectives, activities, and evaluations to meet that need, using either small group or modeling strategies
   D. Write scripts or collect materials to use in modeling training for a specific socially acceptable behavior
   E. In a sociodrama or simulation, respond to maladaptive behaviors using the intervention strategies in sequential or nearly sequential order, naming them as they are used
   F. Write a script or make a tape (video or audio) in which are illustrated at least four ways of talking to others that preserve their dignity and show respect

LESSON PLAN, SESSION 1: MALADAPTIVE BEHAVIORS

Competencies: I (A): Trainees will know and be able to discuss what maladaptive behaviors are, giving examples, and how they are counterproductive

    I (B): Trainees will know and be able to discuss some physiological, social, and personal explanations for maladaptive behaviors in older DD adults

    II (A): Trainees will be able to identify maladaptive behaviors

Objectives: I (A): After discussion, trainees will list at least eight maladaptive behaviors and tell how they are annoying, counterproductive, or harmful to others

    I (B): After instruction, trainees will list possible causes of maladaptive behavior in these categories: physiological, learned, psychological, and social

    II (A): In either a simulated situation or viewing a videotape, trainees will be able to identify maladaptive behaviors when they are displayed

Instructor	Trainee	Materials
Present introduction to concept of discipline with dignity (Lecture Outline 1.I, 1.IIA–B)	Take notes or underline text	Primary text, Overview, Section IV; Chapter 13
Ask questions to clarify understanding: Why is punishment counter-productive? What behaviors are not the subject of this training?	Respond to questions	Chalkboard and/or flipchart Chalk or marker
Introspection: "Remember a time in school when a student in your class was severely disciplined. Think about how you felt. How did the class react to the incident?"	Think about the suggested event from school days; tell the group, if desired.	

(continued)

LESSON PLAN, SESSION 1: MALADAPTIVE BEHAVIORS *(continued)*

Instructor	Trainee	Materials
Discuss categories of maladaptive behavior (Lecture Outline 1.IIC, D); distribute Handout 1: "Maladaptive Behaviors"	Discuss	Handout 1: "Maladaptive Behaviors"
Refer trainees to Handout 1; ask if any of the behaviors are unique to people with developmental disabilities:		
Are there any of the behaviors the trainees have never done themselves?		
How do others react when nonhandi-capped people act maladaptively?		
Lead discussion on "Why are mal-adaptive behaviors more tolerated in normal people than in MR/DD or old people?" (Lecture Outline 1.IIE)	Discuss question	
Discuss possible causes of maladaptive behavior (Lecture Outline 1.III); distribute Handout 2: "Behind the Behaviors"	Take notes or underline text	Handout 2: "Behind the Behaviors"
Have the trainees form pairs; distribute Activity Handout 1: "Powerlessness"	Participate in dyad; report and discuss findings	Activity Handout 1: "Powerlessness"
Summarize "powerlessness" as ultimate frustration (common denominators from dyad reports)		

Evaluation: Give group these headings: "Physiological," "Psychological," and "Social"; have them list as many possible causes of mal-adaptive behavior under each heading as they can remember from the lecture

LECTURE OUTLINE 1: INTRODUCTION AND MALADAPTIVE BEHAVIOR

I. Philosophy
   A. Working with dependent adults in ways that will
      1. Prevent maladaptive behaviors
      2. Correct maladaptive behaviors
      3. Preserve the dignity of the person
      4. Enhance self-esteem
      5. Special techniques needed for severe behavior disorders
   B. Role of professional, family member, or other caregiver as
      1. Leader
      2. Facilitator
      3. Cooperator
      4. Teacher
   C. Importance of caregiver attitudes in working with dependent adults, such as
      1. Nonthreatening
      2. Understanding/empathetic
      3. Adult-to-adult, nonpatronizing
II. Definitions
   A. "Dependent adults" within the context of this presentation are persons who rely upon others for much of their care, including
      1. Persons who live semi-independently, in foster homes, group homes, nursing homes
      2. "Frail" elderly
      3. Developmentally disabled persons
   B. "Leader" as used in this book refers to anyone who has care of dependent adults, including teacher, habilitation staff, workshop supervisor, guardian/family member, direct care staff; refers to person who is assisting the individual to overcome unwanted behaviors
   C. "Maladaptive behaviors" are those that are inappropriate in a social context
      1. Annoying to others
      2. Have an adverse effect upon others
      3. Are counterproductive in individual's life course
   D. Types of maladaptive behaviors
      1. Passive annoying behaviors
      2. Active annoying behaviors
      3. Those that affect others adversely
   E. Reactions of others to maladaptive behaviors
      1. Tendency to overlook or consider just a passing behavior in nonhandicapped person because of his/her valued position
      2. Possible attitude that maladaptive behaviors are one aspect of retardation
III. Possible causes of maladaptive behaviors
   A. Physiological causes
      1. Pain
         a. Headache
         b. Foot discomfort
         c. Toothache
         d. Other minor/major bodily discomfort

    2.   Sensory changes
        a.   Hearing loss
        b.   Loss of vision
        c.   Reduction in sense of smell, taste
    3.   Simple distresses
        a.   Hunger
        b.   Thirst
        c.   Uncomfortable position
        d.   Room temperature
    4.   Sexual tension
    5.   Neurological trauma resulting in
        a.   Random movement
        b.   Uncontrollable movement
        c.   Profanity
        d.   Repetitious noise making
    6.   Limitations of ability for verbal expression
    7.   Importance of physical checkup
B.   Psychological causes
    1.   Low self-esteem
    2.   Anger
    3.   Need for love and caring
    4.   Grieving, due to loss
    5.   Feelings of inadequacy
C.   Social causes
    1.   Frustration due to
        a.   Poor verbal skills
        b.   Limited repertoire of appropriate responses
        c.   Limited ability to interpret social feedback
    2.   Powerlessness
    3.   Feelings of being deprived, victimized
    4.   Need for acceptance, recognition
    5.   Need for security, reassurance
    6.   Loss
    7.   Lack of stimulation in the environment
D.   Learned behaviors due to
    A.   Institutionalization
    B.   Poor example set by leader/caregiver
    C.   Boredom
    D.   Reinforcement of negative behavior

MALADAPTIVE BEHAVIORS

Passive Annoying Behaviors

Glaring

Refusing tasks

Delaying

Rocking

Stalling

Not eating

Not answering

Refusing food

Moving slowly

Muttering

Feigning sleep

Not shaving

Displaying fear

Pouting

Not cooperating

Moving around constantly

Never finishing projects

Not speaking to others

Talking to oneself

Ignoring environment

Isolating self

Refusing to make decisions

Being apathetic

Dressing carelessly

Dressing very inappropriately

Seeming totally passive

Denying anything is wrong

Forgetting things often

Active Annoying Behaviors

Pacing

Name calling

Griping

Wandering

Whining

Complaining

Crying a lot

Ignoring danger

Using profanity

Talking loudly

Interrupting

Speaking rudely, snappishly

Making repetitious noise

Frequently going off task

Constantly dropping things

Strewing things around

Losing things often

Laughing inappropriately

Repeating a request excessively

Showing resentment

Exaggerating

Behaviors that Affect Self and Others Adversely

Pushing

Shoving

Grabbing

Hitting

Name calling

Throwing things

Mocking

Arguing

Blaming

Running away

Screaming, yelling

Damaging property

Inappropriate sexual approach

Stealing

Cursing

Kicking

Dominating

Breaking

Threatening

Self-injurious behaviors

BEHIND THE BEHAVIORS

Some considerations about causes of maladaptive behaviors in dependent and older adults

Physiological

Chronic conditions: arthritis, diabetes, circulatory or heart disease, foot problems, aching teeth, poorly fitting dentures, backache, low energy

Temporary problems: stomachache, toothache, headcold, headache, fatigue, menstrual cramps, nervousness

Sensory changes: blurring of vision, difficulty hearing, lessening of taste perceptions

Discomforts: hunger, thirst, need to void, chill or heat, uncomfortable chair, need to move around after too much sitting, sexual tension

Neurological: Alzheimer symptoms (forgetting, inability to interpret what is said, aphasia), uncontrollable movements or talk, mental illness

Learned Behaviors

Institutional: self-stimulation, repetitious talk or pacing, nonsense babbling, withdrawal, verbal or physical aggression

Related to experience: learned helplessness, passivity, aggressiveness

Reaction to frustration: poor verbal skills, inability to reason or win arguments, communication problems, inability to express wants and needs, slow responses, feeling of powerlessness

Loss: family members dead or far away or not interested, changes in residence (loss of caring friends, staff), possessions taken or lost, physical losses, loss of meaningful activity, loss of life roles (either those once held or never experienced)

Low self-esteem: society reacts to noncontributors, adults with MR/DD have few accomplishments, possibly don't look good, feel unloved, unwanted, useless, devalued

POWERLESSNESS

1. Remember a time your family moved or someone you cared a lot about moved away. Or remember how you felt when you left home for a new situation—away from those who loved you. How did it feel to lose old contacts and supports?

2. Think about situations in your life when you felt powerless to change the way things were done. Maybe the situation involved something that was done to you that you couldn't stop or control (sitting in a dentist's chair, having a baby, being in the military service, for example). How did you feel? Did it affect your behavior?

3. Recall an experience you had of feeling low self-esteem (when you failed a test, when your love affair ended, when you were left out of a party). How did it feel? Did it affect your behavior? How would it have been if you had no compensating things about yourself to feel good about?

LESSON PLAN, SESSION 2: PREVENTION

Competencies: I (C): Trainees will know and be able to discuss some environmental changes that can be made to prevent occurrences of maladaptive behaviors

I (D): Trainees will know and be able to discuss recommended training methods for teaching socially acceptable behaviors and practicing them

II (B): Trainees will be able to make a checklist to evaluate an environment

II (C): Trainees will be able to design a plan with objectives and activities for a group meeting of dependent adults

II (D): Trainees will be able to develop a model of instruction in socially acceptable behavior using either live modeling, videotaping, audiotaping, or photos

Objectives: I (C): Trainees will describe an instructional program for a group of older DD adults that uses either modeling or small group work to teach a socially acceptable behavior

II (B): Trainees will be able to identify elements in a given environment that might lead to maladaptive behaviors and recommend modifications

II (C): Given the need to train clients in a specific behavior, trainees will be able to prepare lesson plans with objectives, activities, and evaluations to meet that need, using either small group or modeling strategies

II (D): Trainees will be able to write scripts or collect materials to use in modeling training for a specific socially acceptable behavior

Instructor	Trainee	Materials
Discuss environmental considerations in prevention of maladaptive behavior (Lecture Outline 2)	Take notes or underline text	Primary text, Chapter 14
Ask trainees to identify aspects of training site that contribute to or detract from good learning experience; list responses on chalkboard or flipchart	Respond	Chalkboard or flipchart
Ask group to identify feelings, moods, activities that seem to be evoked by different colors, as these are presented	Respond	Color charts (11 × 18)
Discuss working with groups, concept of "group as problem solver"	Listen and take notes	Primary text, Chapter 14
Distribute and explain Activity Handout 1: "Simulation: Group Dynamics"	Participate in simulation	Activity Handout 1: "Simulation: Group Dynamics"
Conduct feedback session with observer reporting	"Observer" report group dynamics	
Present concept of "modeling" as a method of teaching appropriate behavior	Listen and take notes	Primary text, Chapter 14

Evaluation: Have group list environmental changes they would recommend either for the training site or their work site

LECTURE OUTLINE 2: ENVIRONMENTAL ASPECTS OF PREVENTION

I.   Some aspects of the environment, if controlled, will contribute toward prevention of maladaptive behaviors
    A. Color
        1. Stimulating
        2. Unstimulating
        3. Examples (e.g., for those who have Alzheimer's disease, nonstimulating, simple)
    B. Space
        1. Need for personal space
        2. Effect of crowding
    C. Light
        1. A special need for many older people who are experiencing loss of vision
    D. Functional arrangement of furniture
        1. Convenience
        2. Avoidance of barriers
    E. Temperature
        1. If technically beyond control, adjust with more or less clothing
    F. Order, cleanliness
    G. Interest centers
        1. Pictures, art objects
        2. Aquarium
        3. Collections
    H. Level of noise
    I. Smoking/nonsmoking

II. Areas of environment may be differently designed and/or decorated depending on function
    A. Shared living areas
    B. Work space
    C. Activity areas
    D. Personal (assigned room) space
        1. Should be a place for individual expression
        2. May be more "cluttered" than shared space

III. Objectives of environmental planning to prevent maladaptive behavior
    A. Warmth of atmosphere
    B. Serenity
    C. Security
    D. Function
    E. Orientation
        1. Color coding; directionals; graphics

IV. Involvement of clients in environmental planning contributes to positive behavior
    A. "Good" feelings of ownership
    B. Opportunity for choice enhances self-esteem

SIMULATION: GROUP DYNAMICS

1. Form groups of 6–7.
2. Read the following simulation and select roles to portray.

Making a House a Home

The staff and residents of a group home are having a meeting to decide on the assignment of household tasks. The residents are older adults who have just come to the
newly opened group home after living for decades in an institution. They are fairly high
functioning and in generally good physical condition. One is in a wheelchair, and one
has a spastic right arm.

3. Designate one group member to be the observer.
4. Conduct the simulated meeting. Observer note: who took leadership (formal and informal), interactions (resident-resident, resident-staff, leader-staff). Note also attempts to
   manipulate or persuade, group rules, who had the major role in proposing solutions.
5. Report back
   a. The plan that was developed
   b. Comments of the observer

LESSON PLAN, SESSION 3: INTERVENTION

Competencies: I (E): Trainees will know and be able to discuss why punishment is counterproductive and discipline involving decision making based upon choice is preferable

I (F): Trainees will know and be able to discuss the use of least intrusive intervention techniques to prevent escalation of behavior problems

Objectives: I (D): Trainees will be able to demonstrate intervention strategies that prevent escalation of maladaptive behaviors

I (E): Trainees will give at least five reasons that punishment is counterproductive as a way of controlling behavior in others

I (F): Trainees will identify the elements needed for self-discipline as discussed by Dreikurs

I (F): Given a situation where maladaptive behaviors are portrayed in a sociodrama or a videotaped episode, trainees will suggest three intervention strategies proposed by Redl and modified for primary text

II (E): In a sociodrama, trainees will be able to respond to maladaptive behaviors using the intervention strategies in sequential or nearly sequential order, naming them as they are used

Instructor	Trainee	Materials
Discuss discipline versus punishment (Lecture Outline 3.I)	Take notes or underline text	Primary text, Chapter 15
Distribute Handout 1: "Discipline/Punishment"		Handout 1: "Discipline/Punishment"
Present information about intervention strategies (Lecture Outline 3.II–3.V)	Take notes or underline text	Primary text, Chapter 15

Distribute Handout 2: "Interventions" Lead discussion: What is the pattern of increased interference? How does the leader avoid calling attention to the adult? How does the leader remain on the same side as the adult in each intervention?	Participate in discussion	Handout 2: "Interventions"
Intervention activity: 1. Present videotape showing maladaptive behaviors by older adults or 2. Present prearranged live simulations of situations described in primary text (or similar situations) Ask each trainee to write a paragraph describing the behavior and the intervention strategy	Observe the presentation; write a paragraph as requested; exchange with partner and critique	Videotape; paper and pens
Discuss each strategy solicited from trainees	Contribute to discussion	

Evaluation: Class can name over eight intervention strategies.

LECTURE OUTLINE 3: INTERVENTION TECHNIQUES

I.   Definitions and implications
    A.   Discipline
        1.   Self-control, imposed by individuals upon themselves—Dreikurs
        2.   Requires
            a.   Freedom to choose how to act
            b.   Understanding what the results of actions are
            c.   Ability to make decisions
    B.   Punishment
        1.   Physical, psychological pain, humiliation, isolation, or revenge imposed on a person by someone else—Dreikurs
        2.   Why punishment is counterproductive
            a.   It doesn't preserve dignity
            b.   It increases feelings of powerlessness
            c.   It breaks bonds of trust and caring
            d.   It shows the leader's weakness of control
            e.   It causes powerless people to retaliate
            f.   It weakens group belonging—fear spreads to the group
            g.   It reinforces low self-esteem of the person punished
            h.   It models the wrong behavior to those being punished
            i.   It doesn't demonstrate the correct behavior
            j.   It reinforces the lack of ability to out-talk or out-argue which characterizes dependent and underskilled adults
            k.   It arouses emotions, not reason

II. Intervention strategies—Redl
    A.   Praise the desired behavior when person behaves well under provocation
    B.   Interventions that prevent escalation of conflicts
        1.   Planned ignoring (don't take bait)
        2.   Send a body language signal
        3.   Move in closer
        4.   Get involved in what the person is doing
        5.   Show affection or caring
        6.   Give a little help
        7.   Interpret what happened
        8.   Regroup the people
        9.   Request cooperation
        10. Limit space and material
        11. Reestablish self-control
        12. Promise a reward
        13. Use physical restraint
        14. Threaten to punish

III. When all else fails
    A.   ACCESS study shows little severe behavior in older adults with developmental disabilities

B. What to do in crisis
   1. Follow agency procedures
   2. Summon help
   3. Restrain acting-out person for safety
   4. Remove person from group

IV. No one is perfect
   A. What to do when leader loses self-control
      1. Admit it to group
      2. Note that everyone has limits—reality principle

V. Summary
   A. When maladaptive behaviors occur, it is the leader's responsibility to be aware, and to use minimally interfering methods of intervention
   B. The strategies suggested by Redl move from mildest to strongest intervention
   C. Crisis situations require special strategies, which should be planned and practiced in advance

DISCIPLINE/PUNISHMENT

Discipline—is control imposed by individuals upon themselves
      —requires freedom to choose how to act, understanding what the results of action are likely to be, and ability to make independent decisions

Punishment—is physical pain, humiliation, isolation, embarrassment, or revenge imposed on individuals by others for the purpose of controlling them

Discipline strengthens the individual, punishment hurts and weakens.

Why punishment is counterproductive:

1. It doesn't preserve dignity.
2. It increases feelings of powerlessness.
3. It breaks bonds of trust and caring.
4. It shows the leader's weakness of control.
5. It causes powerless people to retaliate.
6. It weakens group belonging—fear spreads to the group.
7. It reinforces low self-esteem of the person punished.
8. It models the wrong behavior to those being punished.
9. It doesn't demonstrate the correct behavior.
10. It reinforces the lack of ability to out-talk or out-argue which characterizes dependent and underskilled adults.
11. It arouses emotions, not reason.

Why discipline is productive:

1. It preserves the dignity of the individual and the leader.
2. It gives power to the individual.
3. It strengthens bonds of trust and caring.
4. It shows that the leader is strong enough to let self-control occur.
5. It increases cooperation because of involvement in decisions.
6. It strengthens group belonging.
7. It enhances self-esteem.
8. It models the desired responsive behaviors.
9. It demonstrates correct behavior.
10. It helps those with lower verbal skills improve these skills.
11. It appeals to thinking and reason, not emotional response.

INTERVENTIONS

Interventions that prevent escalation of conflicts and behaviors:

1. Planned ignoring (don't take bait)
2. Send a body language signal
3. Move in closer
4. Get involved in what the person is doing
5. Show affection or caring
6. Give a little help
7. Interpret what happened
8. Regroup the people
9. Request cooperation
10. Limit space and materials
11. Reestablish self-control
12. Promise a reward
13. Use physical restraint
14. Threaten to punish

Adapted from Redl, F., & Wineman, D. (1965). *Controls from within: Techniques for the treatment of the aggressive child.* New York: Macmillan.

LESSON PLAN, SESSION 4: CAREFUL CONVERSATION

Competencies: I (G): Trainees will know and be able to discuss conversational techniques that encourage cooperation and preserve the dignity of others

    I (H): Trainees will know and be able to discuss the names and some features of specialized strategies for dealing with individuals and small groups

    II (F): Trainees will be able to use the conversational strategies that preserve dignity

Objectives: I (G): In a role play, trainees will respond to statements or requests in ways that preserve dignity and show respect

    II (F): Trainees will be able to write a script or make a tape (video or audio) in which are illustrated at least four ways of talking to others that preserve their dignity and show respect

Instructor	Trainee	Materials
Divide class into three groups; distribute Activity Handout 1: "Sweet Talk"; have each group present 'A' portion of one of the role plays	Participate in role play	Activity Handout 1: "Sweet Talk"
Lead discussion on how these ways of talking affect the person addressed and others (leader, listeners)	Discuss emotional reactions	

Present information on constructive conversation (Lecture Outline 4)	Take notes or underline text	Primary text, Chapter 16
Lead discussion Share a memory or an occasion when harsh words hurt Give examples of indirect speech	Participate in discussion	
Regroup and have each group present 'B' portion of role plays in Activity Handout 1	Participate in activity	Activity Handout 1: "Sweet Talk"
Distribute Activity Handout 2: "Careful Talk" and Handout 1: "Ginott's Techniques"; have volunteers demonstrate, with partner chosen from the group, Ginott's conversational techniques using role plays in Activity Handout 2	Participate in activity, *or* be ready to tell which of Ginott's techniques is being demonstrated	Activity Handout 2: "Careful Talk"; Handout 1: "Ginott's Techniques"
Discuss special therapeutic approaches	Listen and take notes	Primary text, Chapter 17

Evaluation: Each pair writes a brief script to illustrate a technique not demonstrated, and presents it as a role play.

LECTURE OUTLINE 4: CONSTRUCTIVE CONVERSATION

I. Respecting the dignity of MR/DD adults in conversation
   A. General considerations about talking to others
      1. Don't issue orders
      2. Speak respectfully
      3. Avoid harsh, loud voice tones
      4. Don't use sarcasm
      5. Don't discuss clients in their presence
      6. Let them speak for themselves
   B. Correcting others
      1. Discuss the person's behaviors in private only
      2. Talk about the problem, not the person
      3. Use as few words as possible

II. Some ideas from experts
   A. Careful talk—Ginott
      1. Avoid
         a. Ordering, commanding, directing
         b. Threatening, warning
         c. Moralizing, preaching
         d. Judging, criticizing, blaming
      2. These result in
         a. Guilty feelings
         b. Hearing "you are bad"
         c. Feeling not trusted
         d. Dropping out of conversation
         e. Becoming defensive
         f. Arguing and counterattacking
         g. Feeling one is being treated like a child
   B. Active listening—Gordon
      1. Trust adult's ability to solve own problem
      2. Accept feelings
      3. Realize that feelings change
      4. Know that helping takes time
      5. Identify with the individual
      6. Wait for trust and sharing to develop
      7. Respect privacy and confidentiality
   C. "I" messages—Gordon
      1. "You" messages—effect on listener
         a. Cause put-down, powerless feeling
         b. Trigger emotional reactions
         c. Focus on the client, not the leader
      2. "I" messages—effect on listener
         a. Tell how the client's behavior affects leader
         b. Put responsibility on affected person
         c. Promote willingness to change
         d. Show group that leader is human
         e. Provide a model for interpreting own feelings
         f. Help people become aware of how their behavior affects others

    D.   Conversational techniques—Ginott
1. Recognize feelings
2. Describe the situation
3. Invite cooperation
4. Be brief
5. Don't argue
6. Model appropriate behavior
7. Discourage physical violence
8. Don't criticize, call names, or insult
9. Focus on solutions
10. Allow face-saving exits
11. Allow the clients to set their own standards
12. Be helpful
13. De-escalate conflicts
14. Speak about the problem, not the person
15. Don't make personal references

III. Conversational styles
    A.   Indirect speech
1. Politeness through indirection
2. Importance of clear messages to dependent adults
    B.   Needs met by communication
1. Needs are strong and mutually exclusive
     a. Need for closeness to others
     b. Need for independence
    C.   Metamessages
1. Metamessage is what is actually communicated
2. Sometimes delivered through indirect speech
3. Sometimes conveyed through conversational style
    D.   Conversational style
1. Taking turns
2. Indicating interest, appreciation, friendship
3. Variations in pitch
4. Questions that criticize
5. Misunderstandings are common
6. Important to know other's style

IV. Summary
    A.   Careful consideration for the dignity of the dependent adult requires that the leader think about what is said and how it is said
    B.   The leader is responsible for clarity, avoiding emotional responses, and preventing problems that can result from miscommunication

SWEET TALK

Form three small groups. Assign one role play to each group:

I. You are a leader of a group. It is time to put away the materials, wash hands, use the bathroom, comb hair, put on fresh lipstick, or do whatever is needed to get ready for lunch.

   A. First, *order* your group to do it. Don't overdo this to the point of becoming abusive.

   B. Next, give the same information in a way that preserves dignity.

II. Sam has been upsetting everyone this morning. He is talking loudly, threatening others verbally, griping about the activity planned, and generally being a pain.

   A. First, correct him in front of the whole group, making personal remarks.

   B. Next, do it privately and supportively.

III. Carol, an older adult with a developmental disability, is telling you that she doesn't like the party you had for her birthday today. She thought the games were childish and the records were too loud.

   A. First, leader respond to Carol with sarcasm and comments about *her*self and *her* behavior.

   B. Next, use Gordon's "I" messages to tell Carol how her behavior affects you.

CAREFUL TALK

Two people are needed for each role play. One plays a developmentally disabled older adult, the other a leader. The "leader" demonstrates first the wrong way (A), then the right way (B) to talk.

I.   *Recognize feelings:* The older adult is weeping silently and looking very depressed. When asked, he/she says the problem is that "someone" (family, former staff person, friend) promised to phone or visit and didn't do it.
   A.   Message—you ought to know people don't come when they say they will.
   B.   No wonder you're sad. You are disappointed, I would be too.

II. *Describe the situation:* The older adult has strewn materials all around (clothes, books, and papers, whatever is available). The leader reacts.
   A.   Message—You are messy, people won't like you.
   B.   Materials need to be straightened up, put away.

III. *Be brief:* The older person starts to leave the room. When asked where he/she is going, the person replies, "I'm going to the bathroom (office, commissary, store)."
   A.   Leader gives long, *involved* instructions, including reminder to take purse/ wallet.
   B.   Leader simply points, gestures how to get there.

IV. *Model appropriate behavior:* Older adult is engaged in quarrel with another. Situation escalates to loud shouting and grabbing hold of other.
   A.   Leader grabs person and shouts, "Stop that shouting" and "Don't put your hands on other people."
   B.   Leader moves in close, talks softly, and gestures not to touch.

V.   *Do not criticize, call names, or insult:* Older adult tries to drink coffee, spills it. Leader reacts.
   A.   Calls person "a slob"—suggests that client may need a straw or a baby bottle. Don't do this angrily; do it jokingly, and bring out in discussion that even "jokes" or remarks made "lovingly" *hurt.*
   B.   React with cool calm—wipe up mess. Make no comment—or just say "coffee spilled."

VI. *Focus on solutions:* Older adult takes material (coffee cup, pencil, book) from another and claims it belongs to him/her. The two engage in a long dialogue about who had it first or to whom it belongs.
   A.   Leader gets in the discussion trying to get to the bottom of it.
   B.   Leader says "Let's find a solution to this problem." They all discuss possibilities (sharing, getting another) and decide on one.

GINOTT'S TECHNIQUES

According to Haim Ginott, leaders use appropriate discipline when they

1. *Recognize feelings*—Example: "I can see you are angry because you have to have lunch late."
2. *Describe the situation*—Example: "I see coats all over the closet floor. Coats belong on hangers."
3. *Invite cooperation*—Example: "Let's all be quiet so we can hear the movie."
4. *Are brief*—Example: "We don't interrupt."
5. *Don't argue*—Example: Stick to a decision, but remain flexible enough to change if wrong. Arguing isn't fair.
6. *Model appropriate behavior*—Show through example how you want others to behave.
7. *Discourage physical violence*—Example: "In our group we talk about our problems, we do not hit."
8. *Do not criticize, call names, insult*—Remember, negative comments are destructive and separate you from the person.
9. *Focus on solutions*—Example: "I see people are taking things from others. What can we do to prevent that?"
10. *Allow face-saving exits*—Example: "You can stay here and do your work, or you may sit by yourself back at the table."
11. *Allow the adults to set their own standards*—Example: "What do we need to remember when we are using paint?"
12. *Offer help*—Example: "Roger took my nails." Leader: "You sound upset. What would you like me to do?"
13. *De-escalate conflict*—Example: "I'm not going to do this work. It's too hard." Leader: "You feel this work is too difficult. Would you like me to go over it with you again?"

Meeting the Unique Needs of Individuals

The Interdisciplinary Process

COMPETENCIES

I. Knowledge: Trainees will know and be able to discuss
    A. The difference between licensure and accreditation
    B. Five fundamental principles that underlie service delivery for individuals who have developmental disabilities as stated in AC MRDD *Standards*
    C. How an interdisciplinary team is formed, which professionals and others should be included on the team, and how leadership of the team is decided
    D. Specific roles of professionals and staff who participate in the interdisciplinary process
    E. The roles and functions of team members in assessment, placement, development of the individual plan, implementation, and monitoring of services
    F. The process of developing and reviewing the individualized habilitation plan
    G. The cycle of identifying strengths and needs and using them to develop annual goals, objectives, and training plans (task analyses)
    H. Constitutional rights of persons with developmental disabilities: due process, equal protection, and Bill of Rights provisions as they apply in service and living situations
    I. Rights derived from the Constitution, rights promulgated by the State, and rights of clients of agencies derived from litigation
II. Skills: Trainees will be able to
    A. Participate on an interdisciplinary team
    B. Interpret an assessment report written by a professional in trainee's field
    C. Write goals, objectives, and training plans related to specific needs

OBJECTIVES

I. Knowledge: Trainees will be able to:
    A. List at least three differences between the processes of licensure and accreditation: licensure focuses upon minimum standards of health and safety, and is required for operation; accreditation focuses upon best practices, is concerned with the full range of services, and is voluntary rather than required for operation
    B. Name, define, and give examples of five principles that underlie services to developmentally disabled persons according to AC MRDD *Standards:* rights and right to treatment, developmental model, life-span services, normalization, and interdisciplinary process

C.   Distinguish between the interdisciplinary team, which assesses, places, and writes the initial IHP for the individual, and the ongoing team, which implements, documents progress, and revises the original plan

D.   Describe the role and function of the interdisciplinary team leader, in terms of presiding at meetings, gathering reports and documentation, and monitoring the provision of services

E.   Describe the expertise of these professionals or the contributions they can make to an interdisciplinary team: social worker, psychologist, doctor or nurse, educator or habilitation specialist, occupational or physical therapist, the individual, and family/guardian

F.   Tell how the process of assessment, identification of strengths and needs, writing the plan, implementation, documentation, and revision is carried out by the interdisciplinary team

G.   Given a written assessment report by a professional in the trainee's field, interpret the report and state its recommendations

H.   Participate in a simulation of an interdisciplinary team meeting, role playing professional, staff, or individual/family member in a manner that illustrates understanding of the role and function and the importance of interdisciplinary decision making

I.   Given a list of strengths and needs of an individual, write a related goal, series of three sequential objectives, and a training plan for one objective

J.   When requested to discuss rights of individuals who have developmental disabilities, tell or write that they have the same rights as do all American citizens, plus certain rights given by states which relate to their condition

K.   Relate the provisions of due process that must be followed before an individual can be deprived of a right

L.   Describe how clients' rights are protected in dealings with service agencies through information required and provisions for protection against abuse/neglect

II.   Attitude: Trainees will

A.   Express commitment to the interdisciplinary process in working with individuals who have mental retardation/developmental disabilities

B.   Describe ways in which staff or families can be assured of securing rights for handicapped individuals in their care

LESSON PLAN, SESSION 1: DEVELOPMENT OF ACCREDITATION

Competencies: I (A): Trainees will know and be able to discuss the difference between licensure and accreditation
I (B): Trainees will know and be able to discuss five fundamental principles that underlie service delivery for individuals who have developmental disabilities as stated in AC MRDD *Standards*

Objectives: I (A): Trainees will be able to list at least three differences between the processes of licensure and accreditation
I (B): Trainees will be able to name, define, and give examples of five principles that underlie services to DD persons according to AC MRDD *Standards*

Instructor	Trainee	Materials
Discuss licensure vs. accreditation and AC MRDD standards (Lecture Outline 1.I–1.IV)	Take notes or underline text	Primary text, Chapter 18
List the differences between licensure and accreditation; ask if anyone ever went through these processes (perhaps when a school was surveyed for accreditation, or when a group home was seeking a license)	Note the differences between licensure and accreditation; contribute experiences of either process	Chalkboard or transparency and overhead projector
Discussion questions: What might be the effects on staff of seeking accreditation for an agency?	Either relate experiences or think of the effects of both processes	
What might be the effects on clients and families?		
Review the major differences, asking trainees to recite them		

(continued)

219

LESSON PLAN, SESSION 1: DEVELOPMENT OF ACCREDITATION *(continued)*

Instructor	Trainee	Materials
Motivational exercises: List on the board or screen: 1. Thou shalt not kill 2. My family comes first 3. A day's work for a day's pay Ask group to discuss how these principles would affect decision making in everyday events; Have them give examples	Consider life experiences in which decisions have to be made: abortion, war, treatment of illnesses, for no. 1; volunteering, attendance at church or meetings, or working overtime for no. 2; taking sick days, vacation, long breaks, working overtime, and anything related to the relationship of time to work for no. 3	Chalkboard or transparency and overhead projector
Discuss how one of the principles affects decisions in a multitude of events		
Discuss the five principles underlying service (Lecture Outline 1.V)		
Give examples from experience and encourage the group to add examples from experience	From experience give examples of the five principles and the effect they have on what a staff person does in daily work with developmentally disabled people	

Do one or more activities from Activity 1: "Rights of Developmentally Disabled Persons"; Activity 2: "Life-Span Services"; Activity 3: "Normalization"; Activity 4: "Interdisciplinary Service Delivery"

Review the five principles, having trainees supply definitions and examples

Leader's instructions to Activity 1: "Rights of Developmentally Disabled Persons"; Activity 2: "Life-Span Services"; Activity 3: "Normalization"; Activity 4: "Interdisciplinary Service Delivery"

Evaluation: Evaluate understanding through the activities and verbal reviews

LECTURE OUTLINE 1: AC MRDD STANDARDS

I.   The differences between licensure and accreditation
    A.   Licensure
        1.   Required before agency or service can operate
        2.   Requirements usually set by government agency, health or fire department, building inspection codes, funding agencies
        3.   Describe minimum requirements
    B.   Accreditation
        1.   Voluntary—done to see if highest standards can be met
        2.   Results only in the honor of being an accredited agency
        3.   Represents the best practices as described by professionals, advocates, and service providers in the field
        4.   Educational aspect results from staff making a presurvey and self-evaluation of services
        5.   May result in improved services because attention is called to unmet standards, and time is given to improve before the outside surveyor comes in
II. Historic base of development of AC MRDD *Standards*
    A.   American Association on Mental Deficiency (AAMD) major professional organization developed first standards; now called American Association on Mental Retardation
        1.   *Standards for State Residential Institutions for the Mentally Retarded* (1964)
        2.   By 1969, 134 state institutions (90%) were evaluated
        3.   National Planning Committee on Accreditation of Residential Centers for the Retarded (1969) added members from:
            a.   American Medical Association (AMA)
            b.   American Psychiatric Association (APA)
            c.   Council for Exceptional Children (CEC)
            d.   National Association for Retarded Children (NARC), now renamed Association for Retarded Citizens
            e.   United Cerebral Palsy Association (UCP)
        4.   Developed the Accreditation Council for Services to Mentally Retarded and Other Developmentally Disabled Persons (AC MRDD) within Joint Commission on the Accreditation of Hospitals (JCAH)
            a.   Medical model for services
            b.   Prestige of JCAH legitimized AC MRDD
        5.   Membership on council changed over time
            a.   American Academy of Pediatrics
            b.   American Nurses Association
            c.   American Psychological Association
            d.   National Association of Private Residential Facilities
            e.   Epilepsy Foundation of America
            f.   National Association of Social Workers
            g.   National Society for Autistic Citizens
        6.   These members contribute to financial support and appoint members to the Accreditation Council

       7. These agencies represent several classes of groups
         a. Professions
         b. Advocacy organizations
         c. Service providers

III. Process of accreditation
    A. Formal application
       1. Agency may request training
       2. Materials sent to agency for self-survey
    B. Agency self-survey
       1. Given list of standards
       2. Staff rate agency on provision of services in accord with each standard
       3. Agency has several months to bring deficiencies into compliance
    C. On-site survey by AC MRDD
       1. Compare their ratings to those in self-survey
       2. Conduct program audits
       3. Interview public and consumers

IV. Review important points
    A. Accreditation is different from licensure
    B. The standards were developed by a wide range of professionals, advocacy agencies, and providers
    C. The process begins with a self-survey followed by an on-site survey
    D. Accreditation helps a staff learn about the best practices in the field

V. Principles underlying services
    A. Rights and right to treatment
       1. Definition: individual with developmental disabilities has the same fundamental rights as other persons, plus the right to receive adequate treatment and habilitation
       2. Examples
         a. Right to vote
         b. Right to own property
         c. Right to marry and have children
         d. Right to make contracts
         e. Right to free association
         f. Right to read what they please
         g. Right to attend church of choice or not to attend
         h. Right to privacy
    B. Developmental model
       1. Definition: the developmental model acknowledges each individual's capacity for learning, growing, and developing, regardless of how severely disabled he or she may be
       2. Examples
         a. Give examples from own experience
         b. Former attitude that some were unable to learn resulted in denying education; now people at same level are learning both practical and academic skills
         c. Emphasis upon childhood learning denies that adults go on learning; learning can occur at any age

        d.   Denial of habilitation training to severely and profoundly handicapped people may keep them dependent and bored rather than helping them to reach highest level of achievement

C.   Life-span services
    1.   Definition: services must be provided to meet the developmental needs of the disabled individual throughout the life span, so as to maximize human qualities, increase complexity of behavior, and enhance ability to cope with the environment
    2.   Examples
        a.   Needs change over time (these examples are not universal, just trends)
           i.   Infants and young children need therapies to prevent deformities or inappropriate learning
          ii.   School-age children need functional academics and socialization
         iii.   Adults need work experience and training
         iv.   Retirees need recreation and leisure activities
        b.   Developmentally disabled people need more time to learn
           i.   Childhood delays are not resolved rapidly
          ii.   Learning requires more repetition and practice

D.   Normalization
    1.   Definition: making available to developmentally disabled individuals patterns and conditions of everyday life that are as similar as possible to those of the mainstream of society, thereby enabling them to enjoy a manner of living that is as close as possible to that considered normal in the community
    2.   Examples
        a.   Normal rhythm of the day
        b.   Normal routine of life
        c.   Opportunity to experience the life cycle
        d.   Opportunity to make choices
        e.   Normal economic standards
        f.   Physical facilities
        g.   Discuss dress, grooming, relationships, materials used
        h.   Discuss concept of "age appropriateness"

E.   Interdisciplinary process
    1.   Definition: provision of programming for each individual using a thoroughly interdisciplinary approach
    2.   Each profession sees a different aspect of the individual
        a.   Clients have multiple problems, multiple needs
        b.   Treatment must involve many disciplines and be consistent across sites

RIGHTS OF DEVELOPMENTALLY DISABLED PERSONS

Purposes

1. To know that persons with developmental disabilities have the same rights as all U.S. citizens
2. To know that they also have the right to treatment if confined

Activities

1. List these rights on the board:
   1) right to vote
   2) right to own property
   3) right to marry and have children
   4) right to make contracts
   5) right to free association
   6) right to read what they please
   7) right to attend church of choice or not to attend any
   8) right to privacy

   Divide the group into small groups no larger than five people. Have them decide whether these rights are:
   a. Available to the handicapped without question
   b. Available to those who can show that they are able to exercise them properly
   c. Available to all except those who have been legally deprived of them
2. Assign one or more of the rights to each group and ask them to give examples of how these have been denied to disabled people.
3. Have the same groups list ideas for ensuring that rights are not denied without due process.
4. Discussion question: What effects has the "right to treatment" decision had on the mental health and retardation systems of institutions?

LIFE-SPAN SERVICES

Purposes

1. To think creatively about service delivery at different life stages
2. To trace the effects of previous service upon that which follows

Activities

1. List on board or give each trainee a sheet of paper with these words:
   a. Before conception
   b. During birth
   c. Birth to 2 years old
   d. Preschool (3–5)
   e. School age
   f. Adulthood
   g. Retirement
   In small groups discuss the kinds of treatment needed at that stage or the type of services usually provided. Share the lists and then discuss the next activity.
2. If money were no object, how could services be expanded to meet the needs of individuals at each stage of the life span?
3. Discuss the effect of sufficient and proper service at each stage, starting from the beginning, as such service relates to prevention of later problems or preparation for the later stages of life.

NORMALIZATION

Purposes

1. To recognize practices in service to disabled persons which are not normalizing
2. To be able to prescribe more normal approaches to services

Activities

1. In small groups, either using the readings or remembering from experience, focus upon previous practices that were demeaning or age inappropriate. Use Nirje's list of areas where normalization is possible:
   a. Normal rhythm of the day
   b. Normal routine of life
   c. Opportunity to experience the life cycle
   d. Respect for one's desires, wishes, choices
   e. Coeducational programs and staff of both sexes
   f. Application of normal economic standards
   g. Physical facilities (places of residence and work)
   Add these:
   a. Dress and grooming
   b. Learning or work materials
2. Then give examples of normalizing changes that have been or can be made in each area.
3. Discussion question: Why would staff and service providers want to use inappropriate practices and materials in working with developmentally disabled adults?

INTERDISCIPLINARY SERVICE DELIVERY

Purposes

1. To realize that different people perceive individuals in different ways relative to their relationship with the individuals and to their training
2. To understand that interchange of viewpoints and information about an individual strengthens the services given by each

Activity

1. Each trainee is asked to imagine that an accident or stroke has resulted in temporary incapacity which will require long-term rehabilitation efforts. List everyone who would be involved in such efforts, including everyone who has a professional or personal contribution to make. List may include spouse, children, parents, teachers or professors, employers or supervisors, clergy, doctor, nurse, attorney, banker, or anyone else considered appropriate to be on the person's personal interdisciplinary team.
2. Beside each person's name or profession, list the special viewpoints about the patient that each would bring to the team as well as the skills for rehabilitation that each could supply.
3. Discuss:
    a. Would you rather have a representative of the profession or one who had worked with you directly?
    b. Why would it be important to you to have a say in team decisions?
    c. How would you feel if a team member said you were too "out of it" to take part in the meeting?
    d. How would you feel about having private personal things about yourself discussed by the team?

LESSON PLAN, SESSION 2: THE INTERDISCIPLINARY PROCESS

Competencies: I (C): Trainees will know and be able to discuss how an interdisciplinary team is formed, which professionals and others should be included on the team, and how leadership of the team is decided

    I (D): Trainees will know and be able to discuss specific roles of professionals and staff who participate in the interdisciplinary process

    I (E): Trainees will know and be able to discuss the roles and functions of team members in assessment, placement, development of the individual plan, implementation, and monitoring of services

    II (A): Trainees will be able to participate on an interdisciplinary team

Objectives: I (C): Trainees will be able to distinguish between the interdisciplinary team and the ongoing team

    I (D): Trainees will be able to describe the role and function of the interdisciplinary team leader

    I (E): Trainees will be able to describe the expertise of various professionals or the contributions they can make to an interdisciplinary team

    I (F): Trainees will be able to tell how the process of assessment, identification of strengths and needs, writing the plan, implementation, documentation, and revision is carried out by the interdisciplinary team

Instructor	Trainee	Materials
Structure the thinking of the group by asking how many people have served on an interdisciplinary team; what were their impressions of how the process worked	Participate in discussion if experienced in participation on team	
Present topic of the interdisciplinary team (Lecture Outline 1); use maximal group participation	Take notes or underline text	Primary text, Chapter 19
Use Handout 1: "The Interdisciplinary Process" to help group learn to distinguish intake evaluation teams and duties from the ongoing team and duties	Follow the discussion using the handout as an aid to understanding	Handout 1: "The Interdisciplinary Process"

Evaluation: Put the handouts away and ask the group to reconstruct the process

LECTURE OUTLINE 2: THE INTERDISCIPLINARY TEAM

I.   Who should be on the team?
   A.   Comprehensive evaluation team
      1.   Professionals who will assess the individual's current status: psychologist, doctor, nurse, social worker, educator or habilitation specialist, speech or language specialist, audiologist
      2.   Coordinator
   B.   Ongoing interdisciplinary team
      1.   The individual and family member or guardian
      2.   Direct service providers
      3.   Professionals who have a program for the individual
      4.   Invited members (ad hoc)

II. Duties of members
   A.   Assessment/evaluation
   B.   Written reports to team coordinator
      1.   Updated evaluations
      2.   Reports of progress
      3.   Recommendations for modifications or new goals
   C.   Team dynamics
      1.   Elicit experiences from the group
      2.   Some members dominate, others remain passive
      3.   Need for awareness of dynamics

THE INTERDISCIPLINARY PROCESS

Individual seeks enrollment   **ENROLL**

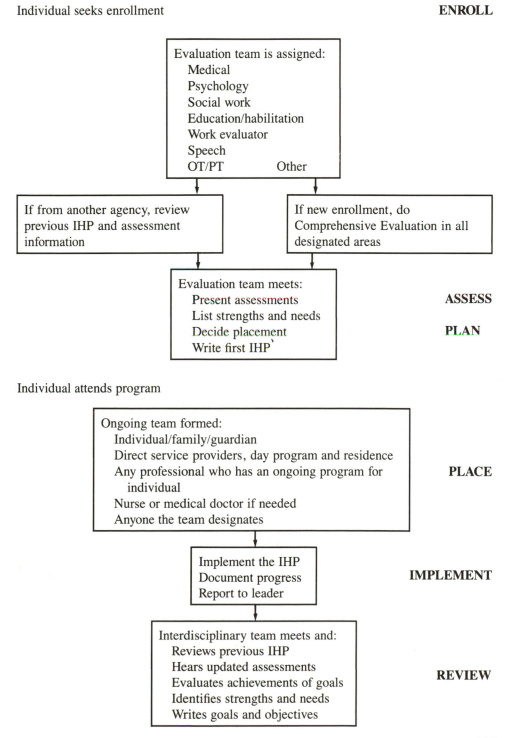

Evaluation team is assigned:
  Medical
  Psychology
  Social work
  Education/habilitation
  Work evaluator
  Speech
  OT/PT   Other

If from another agency, review previous IHP and assessment information

If new enrollment, do Comprehensive Evaluation in all designated areas

Evaluation team meets:
  Present assessments   **ASSESS**
  List strengths and needs
  Decide placement   **PLAN**
  Write first IHP

Individual attends program

Ongoing team formed:
  Individual/family/guardian
  Direct service providers, day program and residence
  Any professional who has an ongoing program for   **PLACE**
    individual
  Nurse or medical doctor if needed
  Anyone the team designates

Implement the IHP
Document progress   **IMPLEMENT**
Report to leader

Interdisciplinary team meets and:
  Reviews previous IHP
  Hears updated assessments
  Evaluates achievements of goals   **REVIEW**
  Identifies strengths and needs
  Writes goals and objectives

231

LESSON PLAN, SESSION 3: THE IHP MEETING

Competencies: I (F): Trainees will know and be able to discuss the process of developing and reviewing the individualized habilitation plan

I (G): Trainees will know and be able to discuss the cycle of identifying strengths and needs and using them to develop annual goals, objectives, and training plans (task analyses)

II (B): Trainees will be able to interpret an assessment report written by a professional in trainees' field

Objectives: I (G): Given a written assessment report by a professional in the trainees' field, trainees will be able to interpret the report and state its recommendations

I (H): Trainees will be able to participate in a simulation of an interdisciplinary meeting

Instructor	Trainee	Materials
Discuss the Individualized Habilitation Plan (Lecture Outline 3); give many examples from experience, and elicit examples from group members who have experience	Take notes or underline text	Primary text, Chapter 20
Organize trainees into groups of six to do Simulation 1: "Reviewing the IHP"; do the simulation through step 3 (steps 4–6 will be done in the next session)	Select a role to play in the simulation; participate in simulation	Leader's instructions for Simulation 1: "Reviewing the IHP"; one set of Simulation Handouts: "Reviewing the IHP" for each group of six trainees

Evaluation: Participation in the simulation showing understanding of the role portrayed

LECTURE OUTLINE 3: THE INDIVIDUALIZED HABILITATION PLAN

I. Process of developing the first plan
  - A. Comprehensive evaluation
    1. Review section from previous lecture about comprehensive evaluation team
    2. Each state has requirements for content of the evaluation; check your own state before lecture
    3. Most evaluations require:
      - a. Physical development and health—medical and dental exam
      - b. Communication—audiology or hearing screening, speech and language
      - c. Cognitive—psychological and educational or work evaluation
      - d. Adaptive behavior and independent living skills
      - e. Social history
  - B. Team meets
    1. To decide placement and program for the individual
    2. Develop first individualized habilitation plan and all subsequent IHPs, which are revisions of the first

II. The ongoing team and its process
  - A. Review team membership from previous chapter and lecture
  - B. Conducting the meeting
    1. Sign in
    2. Hear updated assessments and recommendations
    3. List strengths and needs
    4. Review previous plan
    5. Assign priorities to needs
    6. Develop annual goals
    7. Write implementing objectives
  - C. Confidentiality and informational concerns

REVIEWING THE IHP (Leader's Instructions)

1. Read the following scenario to your groups of six trainees:
    You are the interdisciplinary team for Bill Hossfeld. Bill is 56 years old. He lives in the family home with his 80-year-old mother. Bill works at the Hilltop Industries Sheltered Workshop in the production group.

    This is the annual review of Bill's IHP. Each of you will play one role as a team member. You will have a copy of your goals and objectives for *last year's* IHP. Decide in some way whether the goals and objectives were achieved. Write this in a brief report and give recommendations about this next year's goals.
2. Have groups open the packet of materials and choose roles to portray. Give them time to read the materials.
3. Direct the "case manager/coordinator" to begin the "meeting" by reviewing the materials in last year's IHP from the beginning. When the goals and objectives for last year have been reported upon, discuss the recommendations that the team members presented.
4. If needed, make a new list of needs and assign them priorities.
5. As a team, decide upon the goals for this year.
6. Although the objectives are theoretically supposed to be written by the whole team, have the person to whom the goal is assigned write the first implementing objective, the dates, procedures, and documentation schedule.

Discussion questions

1. Did Bill and his mother feel that their needs were met by the team?
2. How did team members treat Bill and his mother? Did they preserve dignity?
3. Was there good interaction between team members? Did they all contribute to solutions?

REVIEWING THE IHP

Case Manager

You are Bill Hossfeld's case manager. Bill is a 56-year-old who lives at home with his 80-year-old mother. Both are in fairly good health, but Bill is about 30 pounds overweight and lives a very sedentary life-style. He eats lots of snacks that are high in calories and low on nutrition. He gets $350 a month SSI and averages $100 per month at the workshop. The workshop people have been complaining that Bill's production is falling. He frequently falls asleep after lunch and refuses to work because it's too noisy in the workshop.

Bill likes to come to social events at the workshop. He comes to the dances and sits with a girlfriend, but he doesn't dance. He loves to eat out at restaurants, especially McDonald's where he gets double fries, milkshakes, and Big Macs. He is worried about his mother dying, and he doesn't know what will happen to him if she does die. He had talked about wanting to live in an apartment.

Bill is in the high moderate range of retardation. His adaptive behavior is in the same range.

Report

As team leader you have received documentation of last year's IHP goals and objectives. You have also received a report from the doctor, which you gave to the nurse to present at the meeting. You will conduct the meeting, following the document itself and the "Interdisciplinary Process" flow sheet (Handout 1, Section V, Session 2). Be sure everyone gets an opportunity to talk and give their ideas. Be sure the mother and Bill do too.

Report to Case Manager

Bill Hossfeld achieved his housekeeping goal of being able to use a vacuum sweeper. By the end of the year, he was able to go into any one of the rooms in the Apartment Training Area and independently clean the floor. In my opinion he is ready to go ahead with other chores. He told me he wants to get an apartment of his own.

George Erdman
_____
Housekeeping Habilitation Specialist

Report to Case Manager

I think Bill needs to get involved with the exercise class. He came by my office and asked about it.

Barbara Henry
_____
Physical Development Specialist

REVIEWING THE IHP

Bill Hossfeld

You are 56 years old. You live at the family home with your 80-year-old mother. You are both in fairly good health. You attend the Hilltop Industries Sheltered Workshop. You earn about $100 a month and receive Supplemental Security Income of $350 as well. Your mother gives you $35 to spend out of the SSI money. You enjoy working but you are starting to get tired after lunch, and the noise at the workshop is getting irritating. You might be interested in getting ready to participate in a part-time work—part-time senior program group. You enjoy going out to eat and to attend baseball games. You have a lady friend at the workshop who you sometimes call on the phone, but don't take out.

You worry about what will happen to you when your mother dies. She has not made plans for you. You know that some others live in group homes or in apartments with room-mates. You might be interested in that.

You got dentures over a year ago, but you still are having trouble eating and talking with them. You don't know what is wrong, but you often leave your dentures at home rather than feel awkward. Your annual checkup at the doctor's office revealed that you are diabetic and about 30 pounds overweight. You love to eat and are reluctant to exercise.

You are in the high moderate range of retardation, ambulatory, and able to speak in simple sentences. You understand everything that is said, as long as the words are known to you. You probably are timid about actively participating in the meeting. Be sure you approve of the plan, and that it meets your needs.

How did you feel the meeting went?

_____

_____

_____

_____

REVIEWING THE IHP

Mother

Your son is 56 years old. He has always lived at home with you. Your husband left you both in 1945 and hasn't been heard from since. Bill is very large. He is about 30 pounds over-weight. You aren't able to cook the same kinds of meals you used to so you frequently give Bill a couple of dollars and tell him to go down to McDonald's. You know he is eating the wrong things, but aren't willing to argue with him. Bill gets $350 a month SSI and earns about $100 at the Hilltop Industries Sheltered Workshop. You also get a few hundred in Social Security, but you are very pressed for money all the time. You worry about what will happen to your son if you have to go to a nursing home or if you die. You are just a nice person, not hard to get along with, not pushy. You always attend your son's IHP meetings, and you are very cooperative in carrying out any part of the plan you can.

Recommendations:

_____
_____
_____
_____
_____

How did you feel the meeting went?

_____
_____
_____
_____

REVIEWING THE IHP

Workshop Specialist

Bill is a 56-year-old man who has been in your work group for several years. Your group does production work, often using very loud machines to drill or package materials. Bill's rate of production has fallen off in recent months. He gripes about the noise and he hunts out a spot to nap after lunch. You are wondering whether it is about time to think of putting him into a part-time work–part-time senior program group. Another reason he is falling behind is that he is about 30 pounds overweight and hates to exercise. He eats candy bars and drinks soda at every break, and even brings potato chips and Twinkies for lunch. His eating habits are terrible.

Report

You report that Bill's rate of production dropped 10% in the last 3-month period. He refused several job assignments, and was put in a lower group at his request for a few days.

Report that he avoids all jobs around noisy machines, and complains that noise bothers him. He worked fairly well on a sorting job in the other group. You may add anything else that you wish to.

Recommendations:

_____

_____

_____

_____

_____

How did you feel the meeting went?

_____

_____

_____

_____

REVIEWING THE IHP

Nurse

Bill Hossfeld is a 56-year-old workshop client who lives with his 80-year-old mother. He is about 30 pounds overweight and very sedentary at work and home. He eats vast amounts of junk food and always has a snack in his lunch box. You are concerned about his weight. The case manager gave you a report from Dr. Albert Simpson, his doctor at the Doctors' HMO. The report indicates that Bill is prediabetic and needs to lose weight. He has poor circulation in his extremities, and his heart shows the strain. He has high blood pressure.

Report

You will report on Bill's height and weight _____ _____

Give him a blood pressure reading _____

Report anything else you think a nurse would be concerned with. Present the information from Dr. Simpson's written report.

Recommendations:

_____

_____

_____

_____

_____

How did you feel the meeting went?

_____

_____

_____

_____

REVIEWING THE IHP

Speech Therapist (Language Development Specialist)

The client is Bill Hossfeld, a 56-year-old workshop employee who lives at home with his 80-year-old mother. You don't know much about him except what you got at last year's interdisciplinary team meetings. He has been in your adult language development group for a year now. He hates to wear his dentures. When he is without them, he looks "funny" but his speech is fairly good. With them, he is still so uncomfortable that he either refuses to talk or says as little as possible. He did achieve partially the goal of saying sibilants with his teeth in, but he rarely uses that skill in conversation. Decide what you want to recommend in terms of continuation, modification, or dropping his speech goal.

Report and recommendations:

_____

_____

_____

_____

_____

How did you feel the meeting went?

_____

_____

_____

_____

INDIVIDUAL HABILITATION PLAN

3/1   <u>Annual Review</u>   *1986*

Client Name   **BILL HOSSFELD**   DOB *1/13/31*   Sex *M*

Social Security # *216-81-7956*   ID# _____

Program *WORKSHOP*   Residence *FAMILY*

INTERDISCIPLINARY TEAM

Name	Relationship to Client	Agency

Chair:

John Pape –	Case Mgr.	Hilltop Ind.
Elaine Jensen –	Workshop Specialist II	Hill Ind.
Lonnie Adams –	Lang. Dev. Spec.	Hilltop
Linda Rogers –	R.N.	Hilltop Indust.
BILL H.		
Mary Hossfeld –	Mother	

Written In-Put From:	Agency		Date
Albert Simpson M.D.	Doctors' HMO		2/6
George Erdman	Hill Homes	Hab Spec	2/25
Barbara Henry	MCAC	Phys. Dev. Spec.	2/27

241

INDIVIDUAL HABILITATION PLAN

NAME: *BILL HOSSFELD* DATE: *3/1/86*

ASSESSMENTS CONDUCTED, FINDINGS & RECOMMENDATIONS

ASSESSMENT: *Psych Up-date*

Date of Assessment: *6/26/78* Examiner & Title *H. Blackbox Ph.D*

Findings: *upper range Moderate M.R. Adaptive Beh - Mild / MODERATE*

Recommendations: *Training for independence*

ASSESSMENT: *BCP- Activities Daily Living*

Date of Assessment: *9/7/86* Examiner & Title *Jenson. WS II*

Findings: *Self Care skills all independent. Money skills - uses only coins Work skills - attention span decreasing*

Recommendations: *Needs money skills, shopping Possible need to train for apartment living.*

ASSESSMENT: *Speech - Observation*

Date of Assessment: *9-9-86* Examiner & Title *Adams, LOS*

Findings: *Much difficulty with new dentures. Speech skills declined. Needs Therapy.*

Recommendations: *OT. check out eating Speech therapy until speech becomes more understandable*

INDIVIDUAL HABILITATION PLAN

NAME: *Bill Hossfeld*   DATE: *3-1-86*

Based on the Assessment process, the Interdisciplinary Team identifies the specific developmental strengths and needs of the individual and then assigns priorities to the individual's needs.

STRENGTHS	NEEDS	PRIORITY
1) Ambulates	lose weight, get more exercise	1
2) Has all self help skills - Ind.	increase production	2
3) Speaks short sentences		
4) has dentures	prepare for apartment living	1
5) enjoys food baseball eating out	learn money use	2
6) has "girl friend"	O.T. help with eating. Speech therapy - denture problems	1
7) reads all survival words	learn to read	2
	sex education	3

243

INDIVIDUAL HABILITATION PLAN

NAME: *BILL HOSSFELD*

GOAL: *Bill will lose 20 pounds.*

OBJECTIVE	INITIATION DATE	PROJECTED COMPLETION DATE	PROCEDURES	DATA RECORDING PROCEDURES
Bill will distinguish between low and high calorie snacks by June 1	3/15/86	3/1/87	Mother will send fruit/veg snacks with lunch Box

AT BREAK TIMES HE WILL be offered snacks from HOME AND REMINDED OF CALORIES. Document choices 1 x wk. | Record choices 1X WK AT Break

— Jensen |
| Bill will weigh himself weekly and chart his weight | 3/15/86 | 3/1/87 | Bill will go to NURSE STATION EVERY MONDAY before work. HE will weigh himself, STATE AND CHART, AND STATE weight loss or gain | Nurse will ASSIST IN weighing + graphing

— Rogers |

DURATION/FREQUENCY SCHEDULE *Snack 2x daily - Document 1x wk Weight 1x wk*

PERSON(S) RESPONSIBLE FOR TRAINING *Jensen + Rogers*

244

INDIVIDUAL HABILITATION PLAN

NAME: BILL HOSSFELD

GOAL: BILL WILL WEAR his dentures SUCCESSFULLY

OBJECTIVE	INITIATION DATE	PROJECTED COMPLETION DATE	PROCEDURES	DATA RECORDING PROCEDURES
Bill will use denture adhesive and place his dentures correctly	3-15-86	3-30-86	Nurse will see Bill in A.M. daily. Bill will remove dentures, If not in, will wash, put Adhesive on them & place in mouth	1. WASH 2. APPLY Adhesive 3. place in mouth 1 x day — Rogers
Bill will SAY sibilants in words while wearing his dentures	4-1-86	3-1-87	Bill will ATTEND LDS adult class 1/2 hr wk. LDS will provide instruction & practice in group. LDS will document 1 x wk.	1. dentures in place 2. says sentences with "n" SIBILANTS understand-ABLY — Adams

DURATION/FREQUENCY SCHEDULE 1) 1 x day, 2 wks 2) 1 x wk 1/2 hr Training /docum.

PERSON(S) RESPONSIBLE FOR TRAINING 1) Rogers 2) Adams

INDIVIDUAL HABILITATION PLAN

NAME: *Bill Hossfeld*

GOAL: *Bill will be able to vacuum a carpet*

OBJECTIVE	INITIATION DATE	PROJECTED COMPLETION DATE	PROCEDURES	DATA RECORDING PROCEDURES
Bill will be able to plug in + turn on vacuum sweeper	3-15-86	4-15-86	Will instruct in operations specialist 15 min per week.	Plug in adjust height check bag. 1 x wk - Smith
Bill will clean 8x12 carpet using U. sweeper	4-16-86	3-1-87	Habilitation specialist will show Bill how to use U. Sweeper 1 x wk in apartment training class	Above plus Move sweeper to clean carpet 1 x wk -Smith

DURATION/FREQUENCY SCHEDULE   *1 x wk*

PERSON(S) RESPONSIBLE FOR TRAINING   *Mildred Smith*

INDIVIDUAL HABILITATION PLAN

NAME: Bill Hossfeld   DATE: 3-1-86

_____

TEAM MEETING MINUTES: - Hilltop Workshop Conference Rm.

Reviewed 1985 IHP. Noted that Bill did get dentures. His weight + sedentary life style were concerns.

Assessments + recommendations presented. Doctor says weight is real problem. Bill is pre-diabetic.

Last year's goals of reading survival words, discontinued. Decided coin goal needed only practice. Needs identified + priorities set.

Case Mgr. stated that OT services are not presently available for adult clients. Team asked him to investigate possible private OT. services at local hospital. Bill might eat more fruit + veg. snacks if his dentures were secure. Might help weight problem.

Bill said he would try to lose weight but he hates his dentures! Case Mgr will keep in touch about that.

INDIVIDUAL HABILITATION PLAN

NAME:

Bill Hossfeld

DATE: *3/1/86*

INDIVIDUAL HABILITATION PLAN REVIEW SCHEDULE:

90 Day Reviews   -1-86

1-1-86

AUTHORIZATION:

1. Results of the review of the Individual Habilitation Plan were interpreted to:

   A. The Individual (when appropriate)

      (Signature) *Bill H* (Date) *3-5-86*

      By *John Pape, Case Mgr* (Date) *3-5-86*
      (Name/Title of Interpretor)

   B. The Guardian/Family (when appropriate)

      (Signature) *Marry Hossfeld* (Date) *3-1-86*

      (Signature)_____(Date)

      By *John Pape Case Mgr* (Date) *3-1-86*
      (Name/Title of Interpretor)

2. Following a thorough explanation and discussion of this Individual Habilitation Plan, we the undersigned hereby express our agreement with the IHP as written:

   _____*Bill H*_____   _____
   Individual's Signature   Date

   _____*Marry Hossfeld*_____   _____
   Individual's Signature   Date

   _____
   Relationship to Individual

248

LESSON PLAN, SESSION 4: IMPLEMENTING THE PLAN

Competencies: I (G): Trainees will know and be able to discuss the cycle of identifying strengths and needs and using them to develop annual goals, objectives, and training plans (task analyses)

II (C): Trainees will be able to write goals, objectives, and training plans related to specific needs

Objectives: I (I): Given a list of strengths and needs of an individual, trainees will be able to write a related goal, series of three sequential objectives, and a training plan for one objective

Instructor	Trainee	Materials
Discuss implementing the IHP (Lecture Outline 4), taking time to give examples in as many areas as possible; be sure that the relationship between assessment, identifying strengths, and needs and goal writing are shown	Take notes or underline text	Primary text, Chapter 20
Organize into groups of 6 as previously; complete Simulation 1: "Reviewing the IHP," steps 4–6 (from previous session)	Participate in simulation	Leader's instructions for Simulation 1: "Reviewing the IHP"; one set of Simulation Handout: "Reviewing the IHP" for each group
Have group do Activity 1: "Priority 1 Need for Nancy Drosten" individually, and then exchange papers and critique each other's work	Develop a long-range goal, at least three sequential objectives and a training plan (task analysis) for one objective	Activity Handout 1: "Priority 1 Need for Nancy Drosten"

Evaluation: Critiques and rewriting of parts of sequence that need improvement (instructor checks)

LECTURE OUTLINE 4: IMPLEMENTING THE IHP

I.   Writing goals
  A.   Goals describe general direction of training
       1.   In terms of increased abilities expected of learner
       2.   In positive, not negative language
       3.   Broadly enough to cover whole year's work
  B.   Objectives
       1.   Name of individual
       2.   Specific behavior, skill, or ability
       3.   Conditions under which behavior will be exhibited
       4.   Criterion for evaluating performance
       5.   Target date for accomplishment
  C.   Task analysis
       1.   Breaking the task into component steps
       2.   This is the preferred mode for teaching individuals who have great difficulty learning complex tasks
       3.   Give examples (e.g., primary text, p. 191)
       4.   Forward/backward chaining
  D.   Review and put together
       1.   Goals are general behavioral statements indicating general direction of training
       2.   Objectives specify the results of instruction in terms of what the student will be able to do
       3.   The task analysis specifies the steps that will be taken in performing the task to be learned
       4.   Put together they provide a very specific training method that is the most likely to assure learning

PRIORITY 1 NEED FOR NANCY DROSTEN

Nancy (age 55) needs to learn to wash dishes at the group home

1. Write a goal expressing 1 year's progress for this need:

    _____

2. Write three objectives to meet the goal:

    a. _____

    _____

    b. _____

    _____

    c. _____

    _____

    Critique:

    _____

    _____

    _____

Now develop a training plan by writing a *task analysis* of one objective. Use the back of this paper to write the sequence. Indicate whether you would use *forward* or *backward* chaining. Have the instructor review your paper.

LESSON PLAN, SESSION 5: RIGHTS

Competencies: I (H): Trainees will know and be able to discuss constitutional rights of persons with DD

I (I): Trainees will know and be able to discuss rights derived from the Constitution, rights promulgated by the state, and rights of clients of agencies derived from litigation

Objectives: I (J): When requested to discuss rights of individuals who have developmental disabilities trainees will be able to tell or write that they have the same rights as do all American citizens, plus certain rights given by states which relate to their condition

I (K): Trainees will be able to relate the provisions of due process that must be followed before an individual can be deprived of a right

I (L): Trainees will be able to describe how clients' rights are protected in dealings with service agencies through information required and provisions for protection against abuse/neglect

Instructor	Trainee	Materials
Set the stage by asking the question, "What was life like for MR/DD people before their rights were established?"	Contribute to discussion of earlier days of mental retardation services	
Discuss rights of DD persons under the law (Lecture Outline 5); stop for discussion with each section	Take notes or underline text; participate in discussions	Primary text, Chapter 21
Distribute Activity Handout 1: "Rights vs. Barriers"	Participate in activity and discussions	Activity Handout 1: "Rights vs. Barriers"

Evaluation: Verbally review the main points of the lesson, eliciting the rights from the group

LECTURE OUTLINE 5: RIGHTS OF THE DEVELOPMENTALLY DISABLED PERSON

I. Historic background
   A. Past "warehousing" and denial of rights
      1. In institutions
      2. Exclusion from schools
      3. Medical model—no habilitation required
   B. Litigation
      1. Sparked by organization of Association for Retarded Children in the 1950s; lobbying and securing services
      2. PARC v. Pennsylvania
      3. Wyatt v. Stickney (Partlow)
         a. Right to treatment principle
         b. Minimum staffing ratios
         c. Residents' protections
         d. Safe, secure environment
         e. Individual habilitation plans
         f. Least restrictive environment
      4. Willowbrook
         a. Freedom from cruel and unusual punishment
         b. Major part of day in rehabilitation activities
         c. Indoor and outdoor recreation
         d. Medical and dental care
         e. No: isolation, restraints without doctor order, corporal punishment, medical experimentation
II. Constitutional rights
   A. Equal protection (14th amendment)
      1. No one can be deprived of rights because of group membership, sex, race, age, nationality, handicap
      2. Services must be provided to all equally
   B. Due process (14th amendment)
      1. Persons cannot be deprived of or limited in rights without having due process observed
      2. Notification
      3. Hearing with witnesses, right to experts and own witnesses
      4. Rights to review of decisions
   C. Bill of rights (amendments 1–10) (discuss applications to MR/DD)
      1. Freedom of religion
      2. Free speech
      3. Freedom of association
      4. Personal security (free from searches)
      5. Rights in criminal justice system
      6. Freedom from cruel or unusual punishment
   D. Other
      1. Right to vote
      2. Pursuit of happiness
      3. Manage own money, property rights
      4. Privacy (confidentiality)

III.   Other rights
    A.   Equal educational opportunity (P.L. 94-142)
    B.   Equal employment opportunity
    C.   Least restrictive alternative
IV.   Rights of agency clients (as presented by ACDD)
    A.   Informing families and clients
    B.   Abuse and neglect prevention and information
    C.   Committee monitoring of behavior management and agency practices
        1.   Behavior management committee
        2.   Human rights committee
    D.   Financial rights
    E.   Rights to receive visitors
V.   Advocacy
    A.   Agency advocacy
    B.   Personal advocacy
    C.   Self-advocacy

Summary

Persons who have developmental disabilities have the same rights as all other citizens; these rights cannot be limited or taken away without due process; individuals are entitled to individual considerations in this respect, that is, they cannot be deprived of rights or denied them because of their handicap alone; each case must be considered individually

In addition to the rights all citizens have, individuals with developmental disabilities who are served by agencies have special rights to treatment using an Individual Habilitation Plan, to be safe and secure, and not to be subjected to unmonitored punishment; specific procedures to safeguard rights have been established

RIGHTS VS. BARRIERS

Individually, in pairs, or in small groups consider each of these rights and then fill in the matrix.

Right	Source	Barriers for MR/DD
Equal employment opportunity		
Right to privacy		
Right to marry and procreate		
Due process		
Freedom from cruel punishment		
Freedom of religion		
Least restrictive environment		
Free association		
Freedom from abuse		

Look at the barriers listed. What can you or society do to remove the barriers?

_____

_____

_____

_____

_____